Pandemics, Publics, and Narrative

Explorations in Narrative Psychology

Mark Freeman
Series Editor

Books in The Series
Narrative Imagination and Everyday Life
Molly Andrews

Decolonizing Psychology: Globalization, Social Justice, and Indian Youth Identities
Sunil Bhatia

Beyond the Archive: Memory, Narrative, and the Autobiographical Process
Jens Brockmeier

Speaking of Violence
Sara Cobb

Not in My Family: German Memory and Responsibility after the Holocaust
Roger Frie

Entangled Narratives: Collaborative Storytelling and the Re-Imagining of Dementia
Lars-Christer Hydén

Narratives of Positive Aging: Seaside Stories
Amia Lieblich

The Ethics of Storytelling: Narrative Hermeneutics, History, and the Possible
Hanna Meretoja

Rethinking Thought: Inside the Minds of Creative Scientists and Artists
Laura Otis

The Narrative Complexity of Ordinary Life: Tales from the Coffee Shop
William L. Randall

A New Narrative for Psychology
Brian Schiff

Life and Narrative: The Risks and Responsibilities of Storying Experience
Brian Schiff, A. Elizabeth McKim, and Sylvie Patron

Words and Wounds: Narratives of Exile
Sean Akerman

Pandemics, Publics, and Narrative

MARK DAVIS AND DAVINA LOHM

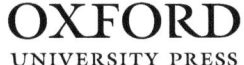

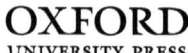

Oxford University Press is a department of the University of Oxford. It furthers
the University's objective of excellence in research, scholarship, and education
by publishing worldwide. Oxford is a registered trade mark of Oxford University
Press in the UK and certain other countries.

Published in the United States of America by Oxford University Press
198 Madison Avenue, New York, NY 10016, United States of America.

© Oxford University Press 2020

All rights reserved. No part of this publication may be reproduced, stored in
a retrieval system, or transmitted, in any form or by any means, without the
prior permission in writing of Oxford University Press, or as expressly permitted
by law, by license, or under terms agreed with the appropriate reproduction
rights organization. Inquiries concerning reproduction outside the scope of the
above should be sent to the Rights Department, Oxford University Press, at the
address above.

You must not circulate this work in any other form
and you must impose this same condition on any acquirer.

Library of Congress Cataloging-in-Publication Data
Names: Davis, Mark (Mark David McGregor), author. | Lohm, Davina, author.
Title: Pandemics, publics, and narrative / Mark Davis and Davina Lohm.
Description: New York, NY : Oxford University Press, [2020] |
Includes bibliographical references and index.
Identifiers: LCCN 2019032568 (print) | LCCN 2019032569 (ebook) |
ISBN 9780190683764 (hardback) | ISBN 9780190683788 (epub) |
ISBN 9780190683771 (updf) | ISBN 9780190683795 (online)
Subjects: LCSH: Influenza Epidemic, 2009-2010—Personal narratives. |
H1N1 influenza. | Epidemics. | Public health.
Classification: LCC RA644.I6 D37 2020 (print) | LCC RA644.I6 (ebook) |
DDC 614.5/18—dc23
LC record available at https://lccn.loc.gov/2019032568
LC ebook record available at https://lccn.loc.gov/2019032569

Contents

Acknowledgments — vii

1. Introduction — 1
2. Pandemic Tales — 22
3. "Be Alert, Not Alarmed!" — 46
4. Contagion — 72
5. Immunity — 96
6. Vulnerabilities — 119
7. News Media Hype? — 146
8. "The Boy Who Cried Wolf" and Other Post-Trust Stories — 164
9. Conclusion — 188

Appendix 1: Participants Who Appear in the Text, with References to Relevant Chapters — 205
Index — 207

Acknowledgments

The research for this book was supported by an Australia Research Council Discovery Project grant (DP11010181) with additional funding from Monash University and Glasgow Caledonian University. We are grateful to our colleagues Paul Flowers, Niamh Stephenson, Emily Waller, and Casimir Macgregor, who worked with us on the Australian Research Council grant.

Most of the chapters for this book were written during Mark Davis's Visiting Senior Lecturer appointment at the Department of Global Affairs and Social Medicine, King's College, London. Thanks to our KCL colleagues, Silvia Camporesi and Maria Vaccarella, for making Mark feel so welcome.

Thanks very much also to Molly Andrews, Corinne Squire, and Mark Freeman for their advice on moving our book project into publication and to Oxford University Press for all their help. Most of all we wish to thank all those in Melbourne, Sydney, and Glasgow who agreed to participate in interviews and focus groups.

Mark Davis and Davina Lohm

1
Introduction

How could you know if a pandemic had emerged? A news story, for example, on television or online or discussed in conversation with a friend might be your first inkling. You might go online and search for information. There you might find public-service guidance framed in terms of preparedness for a public health emergency. Other news stories fed to television, online, and elsewhere may attract your attention. Facebook friends might send you messages, and your Twitter feed might become active. Your employer might send out a message to your e-mail and mobile phone, underlining the scale of the emergency and perhaps linking you with expert advice. Health authorities and political leaders might appear in the media, sharing information and imparting reassurance. This pandemic storytelling across media rich social settings is an important theme for this book.

How, though, would you interpret these messages as a guide to action, particularly with so many of them from so many sources? You might understand that it is not easy to know ahead of time how the pandemic will turn out, thus experiencing a high degree of uncertainty. Imagining what might happen and what to do might lead you to consider accounts of previous pandemics, including fictionalized or part-fiction/part-fact materials from literature, film, and television, among others. Understandings of our worlds, relationships, and selves are said to be found in the stories we encounter, make, and share (Bruner 2002). Similarly, pandemic narratives help us to understand contagion, identify its possible ramifications, and take positions and actions, individually and collectively, on the implied threat to life. In the following chapters we explore some examples of pandemic narratives from popular culture and how they inform the social response to contagion.

Adding to this richly nuanced narrative culture on pandemics is the adoption by health communicators of narrative as a method to persuade publics and individuals to take action. This use of narrative has taken form in radio plays, videos, online games, graphic novels, class room curricula, social marketing, and other materials that convey scientific knowledge and advice in what are thought to be the compellingly immersive and emotionally rich

Pandemics, Publics, and Narrative. Mark Davis and Davina Lohm, Oxford University Press (2020).
© Oxford University Press.
DOI: 10.1093/oso/9780190683764.001.0001

effects of storytelling (Martinez 2014). Narrative approaches to health communication are thought to more effectively advise and persuade affected individuals to protect their health.

As we consider in the chapters to follow, in many parts of the globe this turn to narrative was evident in the social response to the 2009 influenza pandemic. This particular pandemic, referred to in news media as "swine flu," was an extensive media-cum-public-health event, the reverberations of which have continued into policymaking, popular culture, and responses to subsequent pandemics, including Ebola in 2014 and Zika in 2016. A major theme for this book, then, is the narrative turn in public policy and communications, its borrowings from popular culture, and its implications for publics and individuals, in relation to the 2009 influenza pandemic and for other pandemics, such as Ebola and Zika.

Another rationale for our focus on narrative and its relation to pandemic threats has to do with the absence of personal experience accounts in the reasoning and application of public health approaches, including those oriented to narrative. While the swine flu pandemic was a global, national, and local event in many parts of the world and a prominent news media story, few personal accounts of the 2009 pandemic have been circulated in news and current affairs, making the outbreak seem distant and outside of direct experience. Yet we know that many of us all over the world were infected and some of us were asked to take action to assure our health and that of others, including those women who were pregnant in 2009. As Catherine Belling (2009) and Corinne Squire (2007) have noted, too, personal experiences of other pandemics are difficult to tell, because trauma may not be easily translated into story form and because some diseases attract stigma and prejudice, leading affected individuals to be careful about what and with whom they disclose (Davis and Manderson 2014). While pandemic narratives are richly nuanced and mediated—as we explore in chapter 2—the absence of personal experience narrative influences the extent to which public policy approaches fit with how pandemic threat to life is lived. This book, then, also seeks to bring personal experience narratives into contact with public policy approaches with the aim of exploring possibilities for a more fully realized narrative public health.

Cameron's Infection Story

To further explain our intentions and approach, we introduce Cameron's tale of what he presumed to be infection with swine flu in 2009. Cameron's reflections on his probable infection come from a corpus of experiential narratives we generated in interviews and focus groups with people living in the United Kingdom and Australia and variously affected by the 2009 pandemic. We detail our research approach in the section to follow. Here we use Cameron's example to foreground the experiential narrative orientation of our book and to point out how our approach fits with psychosocial approaches to narrative inquiry that place lived experience into historical, cultural, and material contexts (Phoenix 2013, Squire 2013). Through Cameron and other examples we introduce over the course of the book, we aim to show the significant contribution narrative can make to understanding how people experienced the swine flu pandemic in 2009 as a global, biological, yet cultured, phenomenon with diverse personal implications.

Cameron, in his 40s and from Glasgow, was an admirable storyteller, and his account was compelling, partly because it was ironic, and reflexively so. Cameron, at first, depicted himself as having been cynical of media stories on the pandemic:

INTERVIEWER: Were you talking to people about it? What did they say?
CAMERON: I didn't talk about it because I was like "Jesus! I don't want to hear!" because I just found it like most moral panics that get created by the media, I ignore them, which was a bit to my peril, which we can talk about later. (laughs) Well, I mean, it wasn't to my peril but I realized it was actually something real, at a later date. But I'd seen it in the toilets a lot, you know, like you get it in hospitals now, you know (mock concerned voice), "Oh, you have to clean your hands!" All these people are getting taught how to clean their hands which I find incredibly odd . . . showing people how to wash their hands. They were in the toilet, they were in the library, you know, they were everywhere. (Glasgow, 40s, No disclosed health problems)

Cameron's talk of news media and posters on hand hygiene are examples of his engagement with pandemic communications and, in a more general sense, personal experience in dialogue with the expert knowledge systems of public health. The narrative approach we have adopted for this book engages with examples like these and assumes that they reflect the conditions of possibility that arise in engagements with media and communications on pandemic threats and how to respond to them (Wald 2008). Attention to Cameron's storytelling and other examples across our research helped us to situate lived experience in social, cultural, media, and material contexts and focus on how individuals themselves made sense of pandemic messages and, where relevant, enacted expert, public health advice.

The reference to media hype in Cameron's account, dramatized through his rejection of the idea of pandemic threat, is a theme on which we expand in the later chapters of this book. But he also staged this rejection as an ironic counterpoint to what came next, underlining aspects of pandemic experience narrative we think are important:

> I was staying at my sister-in-law's, at the time, and then I just got really ill one day. And, then, I never even thought about swine flu, I never gave it a second thought and I was in my bed for 5 days and I was really ill and I don't get really ill and all I did was sleep. And I'd get up now and again and try and eat something and I've never been so ill in my life and I was just sweating and I was trembling and I said "God!" and it was awful and it was really bad, it was a really not nice feeling. . . . Eh, so I went to the doctor and the doctor asked me about all my symptoms. At the time my doctor was in XXX, so I had to wait until I was well enough to go and get the train and then go up to XXX and go to the doctor and she said, "Well it sounds as if you had swine flu, but obviously you've got over it," she said, "but its left you with a chest infection," which shows you the sensationalizing of it, you know, which kind of reinforced my idea, "Why was there such a big panic?"
>
> [later]
>
> I just put it out of my head you know, it was like, well that just doesn't exist for me anymore. Then . . . and then I ended up with it. So then it became real again, way back to really the start when I thought it was interesting, so then it became sort of a real thing for me it was like "Jesus Christ—I've just had swine flu!" and then I wanted to tell everybody! (laughs) I was like "I've just had swine flu the other week there! Oh it was terrible so it was, I was in my bed for five days—couldn't eat, I was sweating, shiteing everywhere it was awful!"

Cameron demonstrated the craft of storytelling through his knowledgeable appeal to the interest of his interviewer and, through them, the presumed audience of his interview. Cameron staged his narrative by initially alerting the interviewer to the way in which he first rejected the hype of the pandemic but then appeared to have been infected and became ill. Cameron is therefore seen to be actively engaged with narrating his experience of the pandemic, which he found to be partly outside his control.

Cameron's way of telling his story of infection underlines other features of narrative inquiry we think are important: hindsight (Freeman 2010) and narrative imagination (Andrews 2014). Cameron relates a series of events concerning his presumed infection and diagnosis from the point of view of having experienced the infection. His standpoint therefore shapes how he tells of past events and he uses this method of narration to accentuate the point he wanted to make about media hype and what he saw as the general, overly panicky, messaging about swine flu. Narration mobilizes these features of experience, providing insight into subjective life as temporalized being, defined by, but not wholly subject to, the past and fashioned in ways that make futures possible (Freeman 2010). Cameron's story artfully created a then-present self who was skeptical about the pandemic and imagined it to be fake news, but who, through experience of the infection, transitioned to his now-present status as someone who had been infected but without too much consequence. This looking back on temporalized transitions entailed in the 2009 pandemic from the vantage point of a post-pandemic present is important for the argument we develop in later stages of the book.

The account is also a useful example of how narrators build meaning across narrative and, more generally, the temporal ordering of signs (including words, phrases, meanings, and images), a practice that conforms to the inclusive definition of narrative we have adopted (Andrews, Tamboukou, and Squire 2013). This focus on the coding of temporality is important for engaging with influenza infection, in particular, and pandemics, in general, since they have a pronounced temporal and specifically episodic character, emerging, peaking, and ebbing away as they do. This generic pattern, perhaps not surprisingly, accords with Aristotle's framing of three-act narrative (Alleyne 2015)—setting, disruption, and resolution—in public and private modes of storytelling.

Cameron's story of his infection marks, also, what is a major theme for this book: the advent of the pandemic as at first and primarily a mediated event and then, for some, realization that the pandemic had become a personal "reality." In particular, Cameron's use of the word "real" signified that the virus appeared to him to have entered his life world, to become not a topic of news media but a personalized, embodied materiality. This event was met with surprise and then curiosity in Cameron's account, portraying, therefore, how his own life had become entwined with the public life of the pandemic. This particular notion that experience of the events of 2009 was mediated rather than "real," as we will see, is an important frame for how people in our research experienced the 2009 pandemic. Many watched the news as public health officials reported on the numbers of infected and affected across the globe, nationally and in their home cities. This significance of mediation is not restricted to experience of the 2009 pandemic. Writing on HIV, global health and media, Cindy Patton has suggested that, "non-face-to-face spaces are extremely important elements of reality, for activists, for researchers, and for people living with HIV" (2002, page xx). Our book takes up this perspective to show how pandemic narratives across media and lived experience came together for ordinary people, in sometimes extraordinary ways, in 2009.

Narrative, as noted, affords exploration of the psychosocial dimensions of lived experience (Phoenix 2013, Squire 2013). Cameron depicted himself as a psychological subject whose experience was imbued with thoughts, feelings, self-address, and interpersonal relations in dynamic process. His account had an air of self-discovery through his storytelling, for example, when he referred to having at first rejected pandemic media hype but then, post illness, had made much of the experience in interaction with those in his social world. Cameron, then, took himself as a subject of surprise to himself, not wholly transparent, and his story can be reread as one of folly and self-effacement in the light of the unpredictable turn that events can take. Narrative, then, can be not only revealing of self to others, but of self to self (Freeman 2010). Cameron's experiential narrative is also avowedly relational (Phoenix 2013). He dramatized his account with reported speech and populated these moments with actors and action-figured mise en scène: his illness at his sister's house, and his visit to the doctor. He therefore demonstrated how stories can be told to make narrators into social beings and provide the means of exploring social responses to pandemic emergency.

Further, Cameron's infection story drew attention to phenomenological openness and resisted, as we assume narratives do, totalizing representations of experience. Some elements of self and lived experience escape narrative because memories are incomplete or repressed (Frosh, Phoenix, and Pattman 2003), because narrative fails to capture dimensions of experience (Brockmeier 2011), or because the structures of address of the narrative performance delimit what becomes possible to express in language, text, and image (Butler 2005). Cameron's story did not close off possible turnings in events, but navigated them and especially the disconcerting, self-confounding experience of his unexpected infection. This open-endedness captures how subjects engage with the phenomenological dimensions of experience, including its fragmentary, contradictory, and unresolved qualities. This openness was especially relevant for us since we did not require that our interviewees and focus group participants convey stories to us in a total sense. We asked them questions to help them reflect on their experiences of 2009 and influenza in general. The interview and focus group texts we present in this book, therefore, have more in common with how stories enter into social discourse (Bamberg 2011), without formal beginnings and ends, as interruptions to discourse or interrupted or both, and always in the making. Our analysis contrasts with currents in the public life of pandemics in film and literature where narrative structures—notwithstanding the poststructural turn in literary expressions of pandemic experience—are more obviously inscribed as total, polished cultural achievements. Dialogue between fragmentary and open personal experience narratives and total pandemic narrative, informs the argument we develop.

Cameron's account of his illness connected, also, with a wide-ranging literature on illness narrative and its temporalities (Bury 2001, Frank 1995, Kleinman 1988, Riessman 2015). The emergence, peak, and subsidence of influenza infection—a pattern that mirrors the public life of a pandemic—is episodic and as the phenomenon of reinfection with influenza virus implies, can recur. Illness narrative, however, is typically associated with chronic illnesses (Dow, Rocher, and Ziebland 2012) or survival narratives among those with life-threatening illness such as cancer (Chou et al. 2011) or HIV (Beuthin, Bruce, and Sheilds 2014). At stake in these accounts of illness is the transformation of subjective experience; how people internalize, negotiate, appropriate, or resist identities and normativities associated with their diagnoses, treatments, and survival. Arthur Frank's framing of cancer survival stories (1995) in terms of "restitution," "chaos," "testimony," and "quest" is a well-known example that connects with a more general literature on ordeal and survival, for example, holocaust survivor narratives (Fischer 2014) and sexual abuse narratives (Naples 2003), that operate across public life and lived experience. Cameron's story—a short-term episode of infection that came as a surprise, which was not in the end officially diagnosed and from which he recovered despite the intensity of the experience—only partly coheres with the tradition of illness narrative and related tropes of ordeal and survival. Complicating matters further, some of our participants had preexisting health conditions, such as lung disease or HIV, so for them both episodic pandemic experience narrative and chronic illness narrative had salience. Further, the pregnant women who participated in our research spoke of the intersection of their pregnancy and the historical advent of the 2009 pandemic, doubling for them the temporalized, episodic qualities of narrative on pandemic experience. We focus, where relevant, on how people made sense of acute and, for some, intense pandemic risk in connection with the *longue durée* of their chronic illness or other aspects of their life situation thought to predispose them to risk.

As Cameron's example indicates, this book explores the pandemic meanings people ascribed to their experiences and the roles played by other people, institutions, and social contexts such as family and work. It counteracts the tendency in public health to focus on deracinated biomedical identities and atomized, psychological subjects to explore the contexts and constraints on how people take action pertaining to gender, resources, obligations to family and work, time management, distance from the pandemic, living circumstances, preexisting health conditions, and, for some of the women in our interviews and focus groups, pregnancy in 2009. This book addresses a specific pandemic event, supplying in-depth analysis, but it also contributes, more generally, to theory on pandemics and their publics and the role played by narrative knowing in healthcare.

In what follows we provide some necessary historical and biomedical context and explain our methods in more detail. We give some information regarding the 2009 pandemic and explain some of the biological and medical aspects of pandemic influenza that made it such an evasive—if anticipated—public health challenge. We give an account of who participated in our interviews and focus groups, and how the experience narratives were generated and analyzed.

Swine Flu in 2009

Cameron's account of his experiences in 2009 points to some of the challenges for efforts to secure public engagements with pandemic influenza due, in part, to its indeterminate but strongly embodied character in lived experience and critical reception of the pandemic news story. The 2009 pandemic also stood apart, biologically and in global scope, from seasonal influenza, which recurs every year and circulates between the Northern and Southern hemispheres. These features of the 2009 influenza pandemic make it an ideal basis for examining the expressions and effects of pandemic narratives.

It seemed to us as if the 2009 influenza pandemic offered itself up to research. Public health systems had only recently developed pandemic preparedness and response plans when the pandemic occurred in 2009. The pandemic was, therefore, subject to a high degree of reflexivity, since it was prepared for and responded to according to these preparations and was analyzed as a test of them. It was a (short-lived) global emergency, but one that was thoroughly anticipated and readily monitored and evaluated, much more than, for example, the global financial crisis of 2007. The 2009 pandemic can therefore be construed as a "reflexive emergency," since its possible contours and effects had been so thoroughly anticipated, rehearsed, and precoded (Collier and Lakoff 2015, Lakoff 2015, Sanford, Polzer, and McDonough 2016). As we explore in the next chapter, a rich narrative culture on pandemics also prefigured how the 2009 pandemic emergency came into public and private life.

The H1N1 viral infection was detected in February by the national surveillance program in Mexico, followed by concern of an emerging pandemic when high rates of infection were observed in communities and in otherwise young and healthy people. The 2009 pandemic began in a governmental sense on April 25, when the World Health Organization (WHO) declared it a "public health emergency of international concern" (2011). The WHO declaration was based on the deliberations of the emergency committee of experts convened to review evidence and advise the director general on the management of the global response. On June 11, Pandemic Phase Six was announced, which was the formal declaration that the H1N1 influenza virus was being transmitted in populations in two or more different regions of the WHO system of governance. The pandemic was declared over on August 10, 2010 (WHO 2011). The pandemic, particularly in its early days and months, dominated the work of public health experts in the United Kingdom, Australia, and many other parts of the world (Davis, Flowers, and Stephenson 2013).

In the United Kingdom, the first confirmed cases were notified on April 27, 2009 (Hine 2010) followed by two peaks in notified infection, one in early July 2009 and a slightly bigger peak at the end of September and beginning of October. On August 13, 2009, the United Kingdom announced vulnerable groups, which they defined as "pregnant women, front-line health and social care workers, and everyone in at-risk groups (those who were at higher risk of serious illness or death should they develop influenza) aged over 6 months" (Hine, 2010, page 2). In Australia, the first confirmed case was notified on the May 6, 2009 (Australian Government Department of Health and Ageing 2011) and there was a slight bump in notified infections in late May with a peak in late July. The H1N1 vaccine was made available in Australia on September 30, 2009 (Australian Government Department of Health and Ageing 2011) with a focus on both at-risk groups and general population vaccination to help curb transmission. Vaccination was commenced in the United Kingdom on October 21, 2009 for healthcare workers and people in identified at-risk groups (Hine 2010). Globally, 80% of those who died with H1N1 infection were under the age of 65 years, in contrast with the pattern for seasonal influenza, where 90% of deaths occur in those in their senior years (Dawood et al. 2012). In addition, the 2009 pandemic presented a significant risk to pregnant women (Dolan et al. 2012, Pasternak et al. 2012, Pierce et al. 2011), especially those in their second or third trimester (Government of Western Australia Department of Health 2009).

Alongside these particularities, the H1N1 pandemic was also subject to the deep uncertainties that characterize influenza, in general. Influenza viruses are, biologically, highly variable (Belshe 2005). People, animals, and birds can be infected with influenza viruses, and genetic mixing can occur within and between species. Mutations of viruses can also occur across the period of a pandemic or over years (Neumann, Noda, and Kawaoka 2009). Influenza surveillance is open to uncertainty since it is based on multiple sources, including laboratory confirmed notifications, in-patient data from hospitals, and the reporting of influenza-like illness from doctors and emergency rooms (Lohm et al. 2015). There is considerable variation with regard to symptoms between people and over a lifetime. Illnesses can result in hospitalization and death but mainly among the very young, elderly, or chronically ill. Seasonal influenza is only rarely diagnosed with a laboratory confirmed test, so most individuals and clinicians surmise infection based on symptoms and knowledge that an influenza virus is spreading in the population, as demonstrated by Cameron's infection story. Symptom-based diagnosis is, however, unreliable. Researchers have shown that self-diagnosis of infection or noninfection was inaccurate, even among healthcare workers (Jutel et al. 2011). Since it is costly, extensive laboratory testing is only advocated in the early period of a pandemic (Briand, Mounts, and Chamberland 2011). The 2009 influenza pandemic was therefore biologically specific but also archly uncertain, another dimension of the challenges faced by public health experts as they rallied to take action and advise individuals about how to protect and care for themselves and loved ones.

The 2009 pandemic's status as a declared global health crisis, its differences and similarities with seasonal influenza and the sheer scale and sophistication of action needed to properly address the emerging infection and potential for death, made what happened in 2009 an important case study. As will become clear in the next chapter, the explicit and implicit uses of narratives across news media, health communications, and the announcements of authorities and experts, underlines the salience of the swine flu case for investigating the pandemic narratives by which we have come to live with emerging infectious diseases.

Our Research Approach

Our research addressed the 2009 influenza pandemic through experiential narratives generated in interviews and focus groups with members of the general public living in Melbourne, Sydney, and Glasgow. The research was funded by an Australian Research Council Discovery Project (DP110101081) grant with additional support from Monash University and Glasgow Caledonian University. Melbourne and Sydney have well-developed though slightly differently spatialized and governed healthcare systems that responded to federal and global initiatives on the 2009 pandemic. Melbourne, in particular, turned out to be an important city in the global response, since it experienced some of the first notified infections outside Mexico and the United States and evidence was quickly gathered of the rapid spread of the virus and its clinical characteristics in the city's population. According to news media at the time, Melbourne for a few weeks in 2009 was the "flu capital of the world" (Wilson 2009) due to the extensive notifications of infection made there. Melbourne is also thought to have been the first city in Australia to be affected by the 1918–1919 influenza pandemic (McCracken and Curson 2003), underlining perhaps the city's long-standing, global communications and transportation links.

Conducting research in Scotland presented us with a valuable opportunity to engage with the international character of the 2009 pandemic. Previous interviews conducted by the first author (MD) with public health professionals and researchers in Melbourne, Glasgow, and Edinburgh (Davis, Flowers, and Stephenson 2013), demonstrated that Scotland and Australia had similar approaches to pandemic preparedness and that, during the 2009 pandemic, public health experts from both these and other countries had interacted, sometimes on a daily basis, to share information and monitor the implementation of pandemic preparedness and response procedures. It has been argued, however, that public health approaches to the 2009 pandemic in the United Kingdom contrasted markedly with those taken in the United States, due to the particular history of the establishment of public health approaches during the late nineteenth-century industrial cities of the United Kingdom (McCoy 2016). Australia's history as a settler society and the use of quarantine in the nineteenth century also suggest particularity (Bashford 1999). Our analysis of the interview and focus group narratives indicated that Melbourne, Sydney, and Glasgow showed more convergence than divergence, though in this book we explore the subtle ways in which factors such as geography and the social standing of Australian public health services and the United Kingdom's National Health Service were reflected in the interview and focus group talk of people from the three cities.

We adopted a community-based method to recruit volunteers in order to avoid some of the selection effects of clinical samples and to ensure that our sample was as diverse as possible. Between April 2011 and May 2012, we invited people to participate through flyers left in community centers and health organizations, public talks in community-based educational settings, and social networking among volunteers. We selected volunteers for interview according to purposive criteria that reflected the biomedical categories of vulnerability employed in pandemic preparedness documents and communications: women who were pregnant during 2009 (or with a new baby); older members of the community (71 years of age and older); people with compromised immune systems and or respiratory illness such as asthma; and people who self-identified as being "healthy" (that is, no disclosed health problems) and who did not belong to one of the former categories. We used these biomedical purposive criteria to enable dialogue with public health policies in the United Kingdom and Australia. As will become clear in the chapters to follow, these categories are entry points for considerable social complexity in the public response. As is typical in qualitative research, we also aimed to balance the number of male and female participants and recruit people with a range of ages from 18 years upward. The methods were approved by the Monash University Ethics Committee, and participants provided written informed consent.

By qualitative research standards, a large sample of 116 people participated in the research in 57 interviews and 10 focus groups (with 59 participants). The sample size, however, reflected the fact that we did the research in three cities in interviews and focus groups according to several purposive criteria. The characteristics of the participants also reflected the challenges of recruiting men, the very elderly, and women who were pregnant in 2009. Interviewees included 14 pregnant women, 3 people aged 71 years and above, 17 people with immune and or respiratory illness, and 23 people who reported that they had no health conditions. We were able to recruit 34 women and 23 men into these interviews. The focus groups included 10 people aged 71 and over, 37 with immune and/or respiratory illness, and 22 who reported that they had no adverse health conditions. As with the interviews, a mix of 36 women and 23 men was achieved and the ages of the focus group participants ranged from 18 to 71+ years.

Actual experience of infection with the 2009 H1N1 influenza virus was, strictly, indeterminate, despite Cameron's compelling infection story and others like it. Seven participants told us that they had had the virus, though their narratives show considerable variation in how infection was decided—personal belief through to clinical diagnosis by a general practitioner—and no one reported that they had had a laboratory-confirmed test, which is the only sure way of determining infection. Further, 11 participants said that a relative, friend, or other social contact had been diagnosed, clinically. As we have discussed elsewhere (Lohm et al. 2015), this indeterminacy of infection lends influenza a layer of uncertainty that is an important feature of the experiential narratives about the pandemic event. Recall of vaccination history was hazy. Sixty-four of the people who participated in our research reported that they had been vaccinated at some time in their lives. Twenty of these people reported having been vaccinated in 2009. Older people and those with chronic respiratory or immune illness were most likely to say that they had ever been vaccinated: 8/10 older people; 39/44 people respiratory or with immune illness. In the "healthy" group 11/47 reported any vaccination, and among the pregnant women 6/14 reported any vaccination.

We adopted a mixture of interviews and focus groups to explore pandemic experience narratives in depth and breadth. The interviews enabled the participant and interviewer to explore personal experiences of living through the H1N1 pandemic, seasonal influenza, and related concerns. The interviews were conducted in a naturalistic, conversational manner that allowed the interviewee and interviewer to explore meanings, check understanding, and revisit important topics. The interviewers focused on negotiating "narrative production" to provide richly nuanced accounts of personal experience and pandemic influenza. Focus groups were held to reach a larger group of people, more efficiently, as is consistent with other research in this field (Hilton and Smith 2010, Holland and Blood 2012), and to encourage discussion of group agreement and dissent on pandemic influenza (Kamberelis and Dimitriadis 2011). Public communications materials and news items were used in some focus groups as discussion starters.

Interviews and focus groups were guided by the same topic list, which was employed and adapted in a socially appropriate manner by the interviewers and facilitators. The topic guide addressed family and health background (household, including preexisting medical conditions, other infectious diseases, influenza vaccination), influenza experiences (including knowledge of pandemic influenza, sources of knowledge, experiences with the 2009 pandemic and seasonal influenza, prevention of infection, hygiene, social distancing, caring for self and/or someone else with infection), public communications, media, and the public sphere (including broadcast and electronic media, public health advice, advice from doctors, workplace, and schools). Each interview and focus group was recorded and transcribed verbatim to prepare it for analysis. The interviews and focus groups were conducted in 2011 and 2012, after the 2009 pandemic had been declared over on August 10, 2010. This lag reflects the practicalities of funded research and is not unique to our research. All social science has to contend in some way or another with the problem of looking back, recollection, and memory, and the 2009 pandemic for many of our interviewees and focus group participants was a brief media event of the then-recent past. The interviews and focus group transcripts were the basis for published articles on topics including engagements with media and communications (Davis et al. 2014, Davis 2017); the mediating role of immunity perceptions (Davis et al. 2016); the experiences of pregnant women (Lohm et al. 2014); the indeterminate quality of influenza diagnosis (Lohm et al. 2015); social contexts of influenza behaviors (Flowers et al. 2016), and the social dimensions of the public response (Davis et al. 2015). Other papers from this research analyzed pandemic preparedness and response approaches (Davis, Stephenson, and Flowers 2011, Davis, Flowers, and Stephenson 2013, Stephenson et al. 2014, Waller, Davis, and Stephenson 2016) in connection with interviews with public health experts.

As we indicated through Cameron's infection story, for our narrative-oriented analysis we adopted the view that accounts of personal experience in 2009 were storied, situated in interpersonal contexts, and in dialogue with narrative cultures (Andrews, Tamboukou, and Squire 2013). We assumed that interviewees and focus group participants were active interpreters of life experience memories but also that narratives were shared and circulated, drawn from public life and woven into accounts. We acknowledged too that personal experience narratives are partial and coproduced in the sense that they were never total and that meaningful experience is emergent, relational, and negotiable. These narrative perspectives are important for social inquiry on pandemics, as they have much to reveal of the culturally situated and interpersonal aspects of lived experience.

We focused on the execution of individual interviews and focus groups as records of social interactions within which narrative practices could be observed. We examined stories and storytelling in the context of the whole interview to draw out subtleties, contradictions, and absences in meanings. We looked for stories and storytelling practices across transcripts, noting how narrators positioned themselves in their interviews and focus groups and the apparent assumptions they made with regard to their interlocutors and, through them, their imagined audiences. We identified methods of dramatization and, in particular, mise en scène, reported speech, and the shaping of protagonists and other actors in the stories developed in the interviews and focus groups. We noted references to popular culture, news media, and public communications and the related mediation of pandemic narratives. We also compared and contrasted interviews and focus groups, to establish nuance, depth, and complexity in the analysis we have developed in this book.

It is common in the field to distinguish between narrative analysis of life experience and analysis of narratives as they circulate in public life (Andrews, Tamboukou, and Squire 2013, Squire 2005). Our approach focused on narrative analysis of interview and focus group texts but necessarily engaged with pandemic narrative culture, which prefigured what people said and did in 2009 and indeed informed the public health address to the pandemic emergency. Pandemic narratives sustain and shape ways of knowing of pandemics, and narrative analysis can provide insight into lived experience and the intersubjective modes of existence relevant to pandemics. But narrative, as noted, is also deployed in public health interventions and related efforts to persuade publics to act in accord with public health advice. Moreover, the imaginative, fictionalized narratives on microbial threat come into public health communications, too. Our approach in this book is to illuminate these complexities.

Our book is of course particular to Anglophone expressions of pandemic narratives and the accounts of people living in Scotland and Australia in 2009. Where relevant we make links with social responses from other parts of the world and to other infectious diseases, including HIV, Ebola, and Zika. Our analysis therefore investigates pandemic narratives through a focus on the Global North, but also establishes its more general relevance, where appropriate.

We have opted to use extensive quotations throughout the book, as these allow the reader to engage more fully with the storytelling practices that emerged in the interviews and focus groups and, on that basis, engage with the circulation and modification of pandemic narratives in the accounts of lived experience (see Appendix 1 for a list of research participants who appear in the chapters to follow). As we pointed out, however, the narrative qualities of the examples we have used do not always conform to what are commonly understood as formal narrative structures. We did not ask people to produce narratives. But we assume, as others do, that storytelling emerges in social interaction and for many reasons proves subtle and provocative for its apparent fragmentation in tension with efforts on the part of narrators to lay claim to coherence. All names used in the chapters to follow are pseudonyms, and identifying details have been left out to protect anonymity.

Structure of the Book

Our book works across different expressions of pandemic culture and its narrative mediations, examining the storied qualities of the public life of pandemics in connection with the experience narratives constructed by those more or less affected by the 2009 pandemic. Chapter 2 considers in more detail the growing significance of narrative approaches to health communication on pandemic threats, reflecting on the conceptual bases for this turn in light of perspectives from narrative theory and biopolitical accounts of infectious diseases. Key themes are the folktale undercurrents of pandemic narratives and also their significance for the individuals who engage with them. In this respect, we introduce Sarah's story of how she realized that she was herself possibly at risk of the virus, in part because of stories on the pandemic circulated in media she consumed.

Chapter 3 examines the keynote of pandemic communications in 2009: "Be alert, not alarmed." A central communication challenge of the 2009 pandemic was advising publics throughout the world to prepare themselves for a possible health catastrophe, but without inspiring panic and therefore jeopardizing effective government. As people in our research pointed out, reassuring the general public that they should not be overly alarmed undermined the sense of urgency that came into the lives of "at risk" people. The chapter therefore explores how our research participants contended with the preparedness message and its potentially contradictory effects.

In chapter 4 we examine how our research participants enacted social distancing as a method for reducing risk. We reflect on the age-old meanings of contagion linked with distance, in particular, the notion that threat emerges elsewhere and in the figure of the other. In chapter 5 we explore how personal immunity was seen as a means of surviving what was seen to be an unavoidable infection and also an individual possession open to acquisition and cultivation. This "choice immunity," as we call it, appeared to trouble efforts by public health systems in the United Kingdom and Australia to promote vaccination, particularly in the collective sense of "herd immunity." In chapter 6 we explore the accounts of people who, due to vulnerabilities associated with their health status and because of coincident pregnancy, had to respond to the pandemic to protect themselves and their unborn children. A feature of this chapter, too, is a focus on invisibility, that is, the ways in which being at risk was invisible to the "healthy" majority.

Chapter 7 examines a key finding that individuals regarded the news media to have hyped the pandemic in 2009. The chapter explains how individuals explained their skeptical reception of the media and therefore cautiously took on their new pandemic risk identities through what we have framed as "persuasion" narrative. Chapter 8 considers how people in our research reflected on the eventual mildness of the 2009 pandemic and how this situation was construed as a false alarm, with implications for public trust in science and politics surrounding world-scale problems such as pandemics, population vaccination, superbugs, and health security.

The concluding chapter revisits the key themes of the book and reflects on them in light of the prospects for "narrative public health." As we will see, a keynote of this chapter is the critical reflexivity exhibited in the persuasion narratives constructed by publics to explain their engagements with the emergence of a pandemic threat in their life worlds.

References

Alleyne, B. 2015. *Narrative networks: Storied approaches in a digital age.* London: Sage.
Andrews, M. 2014. *Narrative imagination and everyday life, explorations in narrative psychology.* New York: Oxford University Press.
Andrews, M, M Tamboukou, and C Squire, eds. 2013. *Doing narrative research, second edition.* London: Sage.
Australian Government Department of Health and Ageing. 2011. *Review of Australia's health sector response to pandemic (H1N1) 2009: Lessons identified.* Canberra: Commonwealth of Australia.
Bamberg, M. 2011. "Who am I? Narration and its contribution to self and identity." *Theory & Psychology* 21 (1):3–24.
Bashford, A. 1999. "Epidemic and governmentality: Smallpox in Sydney, 1881." *Critical Public Health* 9 (4):301–316.
Belling, C. 2009. "Overwhelming the medium: Fiction and the trauma of pandemic influenza in 1918." *Literature & Medicine* 28 (1):55–81.
Belshe, R. 2005. "The origins of pandemic influenza—lessons from the 1918 virus." *New England Journal of Medicine* 353 (November 24):2209–2211.
Beuthin, R, A Bruce, and L Sheilds. 2014. "Storylines of aging with HIV: Shifts toward sense making." *Qualitative Health Research* 25 (5):612–621.
Briand, S, A Mounts, and M Chamberland. 2011. "Challenges of global surveillance during an influenza pandemic." *Public Health* 125 (5):247–256.
Brockmeier, J. 2011. "Language, experience, and the 'traumatic gap': How to talk about 9/11." In *Health, illness and culture: Broken narratives*, edited by L Hyden and J Brockmeier, 16–35. NewYork: Routledge.
Bruner, J. 2002. *Making stories: Law, literature, life.* New York: Farrar, Straus and Giroux.
Bury, M. 2001. "Illness narratives: Fact or fiction?" *Sociology of Health and Illness* 23 (3):263–285.
Butler, J. 2005. *Giving an account of oneself.* New York: Fordham University Press.
Chou, W, Y Hunt, A Folkers, and E Augustson. 2011. "Cancer survivorship in the age of YouTube and social media: A narrative analysis." *Journal of Medical Internet Research* 13 (1):e7.
Collier, S, and A Lakoff. 2015. "Vital systems security: Reflexive biopolitics and the government of emergency." *Theory, Culture & Society* 32 (2):19–51.
Davis, M. 2017. "'Is it going to be real?' Narrative and media on a pandemic." *Forum Qualitative Sozialforschung/Forum: Qualitative Social Research* 18 (1). http://nbn-resolving.de/urn:nbn:de:0114-fqs1701187).
Davis, M, P Flowers, D Lohm, E Waller, and N Stephenson. 2014. "'We became sceptics': Fear and media hype in general public narrative on the advent of pandemic influenza." *Sociological Inquiry* 84 (3):499–518.
Davis, M, P Flowers, D Lohm, E Waller, and N Stephenson. 2016. "Immunity, biopolitics and pandemics: Public and individual responses to the threat to life." *Body & Society* 22 (4):130–154.
Davis, M, P Flowers, and N Stephenson. 2013. "'We had to do what we thought was right at the time': Retrospective discourse on the 2009 H1N1 pandemic in the UK." *Sociology of Health & Illness* 36 (3):369–382.

Davis, M, and L Manderson, eds. 2014. *Disclosure in health and illness*. Abingdon: Routledge.
Davis, M, N Stephenson, and P Flowers. 2011. "Compliant, complacent or panicked? Investigating the problematisation of the Australian general public in pandemic influenza control." *Social Science & Medicine* 72 (6):912–918.
Davis, M, N Stephenson, D Lohm, E Waller, and P Flowers. 2015. "Beyond resistance: Social factors in the general public response to pandemic influenza." *BMC Public Health* 15:436.
Dawood, FS, AD Iuliano, C Reed, MI Meltzer, DK Shay, P-Y Cheng, DBandaranayake, RF Breiman, W Abdullah Brooks, P Buchy, DR Feikin, KB Fowler, A Gordon, NT Hien, P Horby, QS Huang, MAKatz, A Krishnan, R Lal, JM Montgomery, K Mølbak, R Pebody, AM Presanis, H Razuri, A Steens, YO Tinoco, J Wallinga, H Yu, S Vong, J Bresee, and M-A Widdowson. 2012. "Estimated global mortality associated with the first 12 months of 2009 pandemic influenza A H1N1 virus circulation: A modelling study." *Lancet Infectious Diseases* 12 (9):687–695. doi: http://dx.doi.org/10.1016/S1473-3099(12)70121-4.
Dolan, G, P Myles, S Brett, J Enstone, R Read, P Openshaw, M Semple, W Lim, B Taylor, J McMenamin, K Nicholson, B Bannister, J Nguyen-Van-Tam, and Influenza Clinical Information Network (FLU-CIN). 2012. "'The comparative clinical course of pregnant and non-pregnant women hospitalised with influenza A(H1N1)pdm09 infection'" *PLoS ONE* 7 (8):e41638 1–6.
Dow, C, P Rocher, and S Ziebland. 2012. "Talk of frustration in the narratives of people with chronic pain." *Chronic Illness* 8 (3):176–191.
Fischer, N. 2014. "Writing a whole life: Maria Lewitt's holocaust/migration narratives in "multicultural" Australia." *Life Writing* 11 (4):391–410.
Flowers, P, M Davis, D Lohm, E Waller, and N Stephenson. 2016. "Understanding pandemic influenza behaviour: An exploratory biopsychosocial study." *Journal of Health Psychology* 21 (5):759–769.
Frank, A. 1995. *The wounded storyteller: Body, illness and ethics*. Chicago: University of Chicago Press.
Freeman, M. 2010. *Hindsight: The promise and peril of looking backward*. Oxford: Oxford University Press.
Frosh, S, A Phoenix, and R Pattman. 2003. "Taking a stand: Using psychoanalysis to explore the positioning of subjects in discourse." *British Journal of Social Psychology* 42:39–53.
Government of Western Australia Department of Health. 2009. "Pregnancy & H1N1 (human swine flu)." Accessed January 20, 2013. http://www.kemh.health.wa.gov.au/health/H1N1%20Swine%20Flu/index.htm.
Hilton, S, and E Smith. 2010. "Public views of the UK media and government reaction to the 2009 swine flu pandemic." *BMC Public Health* 10:697.
Hine, D. 2010. The 2009 influenza pandemic: An independent review of the UK response to the 2009 influenza pandemic. London: Pandemic Flu Response Review Team, Cabinet Office.
Holland, K, and W Blood. 2012. "Public responses and reflexivity during the Swine flu pandemic in Australia." *Journalism Studies* 14 (4):523–538. iFirst: doi:10.1080/1461670X.2012.744552.
Jutel, A, M Baker, J Stanley, Q Huang, and D Bandaranayake. 2011. "Self-diagnosis of influenza during a pandemic: A cross-sectional survey." *BMJ Open* 2:e000234.

Kamberelis, G, and G Dimitriadis. 2011. "Focus groups: Contingent articulations of pedagogy, politics and inquiry." In *The Sage Handbook of Qualitative Research*, edited by N Denzin and Y Lincoln, 545–562. Thousand Oaks: Sage.

Kleinman, A. 1988. *The illness narratives: Suffering, healing and the human condition*. New York: Basic Books

Lakoff, A. 2015. "Global health security and the pathogenic imaginary." In *Dreamscapes of modernity: Sociotechnical imaginaries and the fabrication of power*, edited by S Jasanoff and S Kim, 300–320. Chicago: Chicago University Press.

Lohm, D, M Davis, P Flowers, and N Stephenson. 2015. "'Fuzzy' virus: Indeterminate influenza biology, diagnosis and surveillance in the risk ontologies of the general public in time of pandemics." *Health, Risk & Society* 17 (2):115–131.

Lohm, D, P Flowers, N Stephenson, E Waller, and M Davis. 2014. "Biography, pandemic time and risk: Pregnant women reflecting on their experiences of the 2009 influenza pandemic." *Health: An Interdisciplinary Journal for the Social Study of Health, Illness and Medicine* 18 (5):493–508. 1363459313516135, first published on January 29, 2014.

Martinez, M. 2014. "Storyworld possible selves and the phenomenon of narrative immersion: Testing a new theoretical construct." *Narrative* 22 (1):110–131.

McCoy, C. 2016. "SARS, pandemic influenza and Ebola: The disease control styles of Britain and the United States." *Social Theory & Health* 14 (1):1–17.

McCracken, K, and P Curson. 2003. "Flu downunder: A demographic and geographic analysis of the 1919 epidemic in Sydney, Australia." In *The Spanish influenza pandemic of 1918–19: New perspectives*, edited by H Phillips and D L Killingray, 110–131. London: Routledge.

Naples, N. 2003. "Deconstructing and locating survivor discourse: Dynamics of narrative, empowerment, and resistance for survivors of childhood sexual abuse." *Signs* 28 (4):1151–1185.

Neumann, G, T Noda, and Y Kawaoka. 2009. "Emergence and pandemic potential of swine-origin H1N1 influenza virus." *Nature* 459 (7249):931–939.

Pasternak, B, H Svanström, D Mølgaard-Nielsen, T Krause, H Emborg, M Melbye, and A Hviid. 2012. "Vaccination against pandemic A/H1N1 2009 influenza in pregnancy and risk of fetal death: Cohort study in Denmark." *BMJ* 344:e2794.

Patton, C. 2002. *Globalizing AIDS*. Minneapolis: University of Minnesota Press.

Phoenix, A. 2013. "Analysing narrative contexts." In *Doing narrative research, second edition*, edited by M Andrews, C Squire, and M Tamboukou, 72–87. London: Sage.

Pierce, M, J Kurinczuk, P Spark, P Brocklehurst, and M Knight. 2011. "Perinatal outcomes after maternal 2009/H1N1 infection: National cohort study." *BMJ* 342:d3214.

Riessman, Catherine Kohler. 2015. "Ruptures and sutures: Time, audience and identity in an illness narrative." *Sociology of Health & Illness* 37 (7):1055–1071. doi: 10.1111/1467-9566.12281.

Sanford, S, J Polzer, and P McDonough. 2016. "Preparedness as a technology of (in)security: Pandemic influenza planning and the global politics of emerging infectious disease." *Social Theory & Health* 14:18–43.

Squire, C. 2005. "Reading narratives." In "Contemporary social theory," special issue, edited by E. Burman and S. Frosh. *Group Analysis* 38 (1):91–107.

Squire, C. 2007. *HIV in South Africa: Talking about the big thing*. London: Routledge.

Squire, C. 2013. "From experience-centred to socioculturally-oriented approaches to narrative." In *Doing narrative research, second edition*, edited by M Andrews, C Squire, and M Tamboukou, 47–71. London: Sage.

Stephenson, N, M Davis, P Flowers, E Waller, and C MacGregor. 2014. "Mobilising 'vulnerability' in the public health response to pandemic influenza." *Social Science & Medicine* 102:10–17.
Wald, P. 2008. *Contagious: Cultures, carriers, and the outbreak narrative*. Durham: Duke University Press.
Waller, E, M Davis, and N Stephenson. 2016. "Australia's pandemic influenza 'Protect' phase: Emerging out of the fog of pandemic." *Critical Public Health* 26 (1):99–113.
Wilson, L. 2009. Melbourne the swine flu capital of the world. *The Australian*. Accessed October 16, 2015. http://www.theaustralian.com.au/news/melbourne-the-swine-flu-capital-of-the-world/story-e6frg6n6-1225724193107.
World Health Organization (WHO). 2011. Implementation of the International Health Regulations (2005). *Report of the Review Committee on the Functioning of the International Health Regulations (2005) in relation to Pandemic (H1N1) 2009. Report by the Director-General*. Geneva: World Health Organization.

2
Pandemic Tales

> .... *it was definitely on the local news every night for weeks. And so that was just like, "Oh my God, that could be me!"* (Sarah, Glasgow, 30s, Pregnant in 2009)

Pandemics make for good stories, so good that there is an argument that they are implicated in the form and force of narrative itself, particularly those that help to bring into being collective life. Gaspar Mairal (2011), with reference to Daniel Defoe's *A Journal of the Plague Year*, has developed the view that pandemic threat, news journalism, and publics form a "narrative matrix" (page 65). A pandemic threat, because it has the potential to affect all, convenes a public who face a shared danger and for whom news on collective threat finds its value. In this sense, public life and the news that helps to constitute it owes much to the collectivizing and newsworthy advent of pandemic threat. For instance, the management of the 2003 SARS outbreak in Hong Kong has been described as highly entangled with news media storytelling (Baehr 2005). It is also important to recognize that communication with publics on health is not a simple matter of coding, transmission, and reception: publics are defined by efforts to communicate with them (Warner 2002). News narrative on pandemics, then, may also be transformative of self-understanding. Sarah's comment, " . . . that could be me," indicates that news stories on the 2009 pandemic linked her life with a global threat and that this moment was experienced as akin to an epiphany of identity transformation, as we discuss in what follows.

In line with Defoe's landmark text, there are numerous journalistic and historical narratives on infectious diseases outbreaks, for example, *Flu: The Story of the Great Influenza Pandemic of 1918 and the Search for the Virus That Caused It* (Kolata 1999), *Pox Americana: The Great Smallpox Epidemic of 1775–82* (Fenn 2001), and *Polio: An American Story* (Oshinsky 2005),

Pandemics, Publics, and Narrative. Mark Davis and Davina Lohm, Oxford University Press (2020).
© Oxford University Press.
DOI: 10.1093/oso/9780190683764.001.0001

among many others. Some storytelling blends fact and fiction, for example, *Typhoid Mary: An Urban Historical* (Bourdain 2001), which dramatizes the life of Mary Mallon, who was implicated in a typhus epidemic in the United States, and *Biohazard* (Alibek and Handelman 1999), an exposé of the secretive engineering of microbes for warfare. Connecting publics to pandemic influenza through first-person narrative on previous events, the Centers for Disease Control and Prevention (CDC) in the United States has published online personal stories from the 1918 and 1957 outbreaks (CDC 2014). Significantly, though, first-person accounts of, for example, the 1918–1919 pandemic (Belling 2009) are rare in public life. As Belling (2009) suggests, the trauma of 1918–1919 may have made sharing stories difficult and, as Brockmeier (2011) contended in relation to eye-witness accounts of 9/11, trauma is itself not easily put into words. Personal experience narratives on the 2009 influenza pandemic are also uncommon (Hilton and Hunt 2011), which is partly why we wrote this book.

Pandemic narratives are found in popular culture, too, and influence knowledge of pandemics and their imagined effects. H. G. Wells's famous *War of the Worlds* has been much repeated and reworked (2005 [1898]). Albert Camus's *The Plague* explored the fate of a city beset by contagion (1991 [1948]), drawing attention to the narrative tropes of ordeal and survival and the related tensions of individual and collective existence under threat. A fictional and devastating respiratory pathogen leading to global crisis was the subject of *Contagion* (Soderbergh 2011), and *The Walking Dead* (Darabont 2010) serialized the plight of US citizens surviving (or not) a zombie apocalypse. This extensive culture of pandemic storytelling, its mixture of fact and fiction and its various involvements in public life and popular culture, reiterates and complicates the importance of narrative in knowledge production on pandemics. Moreover, because pandemic histories, storytelling, and imaginative speculation pervade public life, government, and science, narratively organized pandemic knowing inevitably frames knowledge of a new pandemic (Ungar 2000).

Partly for these reasons, a narrative-oriented examination of the 2009 pandemic is a much-needed contribution to the field. The health sociologist Clive Seale has pointed out that it is crucial that researchers attend to the "culturally available narratives, stories, scripts, discourses, systems of knowledge or, in more politically oriented analyses, ideologies" (2003, page 514) that shape health and illness. Seale argues that analysis needs to bring health, media, and narrative studies together to more ably attend to the complexities of health and illness (2002). He further argues that while the health storytelling circulated in media may seem fragmented and inchoate, audiences can strive for coherence: "People are thereby invited to reflect on the themes of danger and security, good and evil and so on, forming for themselves an overall narrative that speaks of the anxieties and pleasures of existence" (2002, page 32).

As Seale and many others have made explicit, narratives are significant for lived experience of health and illness. Narrative medicine, for example, addresses clinical practice through the stories of those people with illnesses (Charon 2006, Kleinman 1988) or recovering from surgical interventions (Frank 1995). Significant in this work is the importance of narrative for the clinical encounter and the profession of medicine and also to the transformation of identities and lives that come with permanent alteration of mind and body (Greenhalgh 2006, Sharf et al. 2011). Less prominent in the health narrative field is inquiry on infections, with some important exceptions such as Corinne Squire's research on HIV in South Africa (2007), Charles Briggs's and Clara Mantini-Briggs's examination of the 1992 cholera epidemic in Venezuela (2003), Priscilla Wald's account of outbreak narrative across popular culture (2008), and Theresa MacPhail's narrative-sensitive pathography of the policy and scientific response to the 2009 influenza pandemic (2014). Our book builds on this important work to bridge lived experience and the ways in which pandemic narratives help to constitute public life.

In what follows, we consider how pandemic narratives help to make infectious disease outbreaks knowable and meaningful in public and individual life and the related notion that narratives persuade because of their compelling depictions of future events and their consequences. This chapter also outlines the folkloric qualities of pandemic tales with reference to warnings to prepare for danger, affective and moral pedagogy, and the important biopolitical metaphors of contagion and immunity. This chapter, building on Cameron's infection story introduced in the previous chapter, also discusses Sarah's account of the realization that the 2009 pandemic was directly relevant to her. We explain how Sarah spoke of this self-realization of a new "at risk" identity and her acceptance of a course of action to protect her own health and that of her unborn child. Through Sarah's example, therefore, we bridge the public and private life of pandemic narratives, a central theme for the remaining chapters.

Pandemic Knowing

As we indicated in the previous chapter, the connections between pandemics and narrative extend into the ways in which global, national, and local public health systems communicate with individuals and therefore how they make a health threat knowable and advise people to take action. During the 2009 pandemic, for example, public health experts sought to influence the behaviors of individuals by communicating advice on hygiene, social isolation, antiviral treatments, and vaccines (Australian Government Department of Health and Ageing 2011, Hine 2010). In the United Kingdom, communications in time of pandemic were among other matters conceived as a method to "mobilise the population as partners at the response phase" (Department of Health United Kingdom 2007, page 115). In Australia, communications for the general public were conceptualized as methods for allowing them to act to protect themselves and "care for others" (Australian Department of Health and Ageing 2008, page 18) and to participate in the efforts to "protect our country and ourselves" (page 32). As we discuss in chapter 3, public communications in the United Kingdom and Australia featured advice on social isolation and coughing and sneezing etiquette and, after it had become available, encouraged vaccination, particularly among those seen as more vulnerable, including pregnant women. The United Kingdom's "Catch it. Bin it. Kill it." (Hine 2010) public communications campaign encouraged members of the general public to adopt hygiene practices (tissues for sneezing and hand hygiene) as a method for curbing the spread of the H1N1 virus. Public health systems in the United Kingdom and Australia ran information websites for the general public and personnel in the health system. Print, broadcast, and online news and current affairs stories were widely circulated, particularly in the early phases of the pandemic in April and May 2009. Our research focused on responses to these efforts and joins a small literature that has used qualitative interviews and focus groups to explore individual and public engagements with the events of 2009 (Hilton and Smith 2010, Holland and Blood 2012).

Public health communications like those used in 2009 reflect the orientation of the state to the better health of its publics (Petersen et al. 2010). Communications are designed to encourage awareness of and access to public health interventions, for example, vaccine and antiviral technologies that prevent and treat infections like influenza. But communication on a public health concern is also aspirational, since it exercises a vision of the absence or at least the moderation of the effects of disease. Communications on health problems like pandemics draw on the expert knowledge systems of public health and the varied professional actors who operate in this system, including clinicians, epidemiologists, policy-makers, bureaucrats, politicians, communications experts, teachers, and many others. Communications and especially health-related media are a prime point of connection between these experts and publics, especially, it is said, in the case of a pandemic emergency, when the need for information is immediate and events unfold rapidly (Galarce, Ramanadhan, and Viswanath 2011).

The use of communications and media to address pandemic threats is not without precedent and has been shown to bear the traces of the shifting, yet familiar, biopolitical rationalities of the twentieth century. Marc Honigsbaum's history of the 1918–1919 influenza pandemic and the Northcliffe Press at the end of World War I (2013) underlined the linkage of microbial and national threat. Because Britain, France, and Germany were in the final stages of war, their news media censored and minimized stories on the pandemic in the interests of national unity. The pandemic was named "Spanish Influenza," perhaps not because the infection was thought to come from there, but because the Spanish media, alone among other European news media, freely reported it. From 1938 in the United States, the polio research and education social marketing campaign "The March of Dimes"—a term appropriated from "The March of Time," a popular motion picture newsreel of the period (Williams 2013)—included fundraising events where citizens were asked to donate a dime. By the 1950s and after the invention of the Salk vaccine, as Emily Martin pointed out (1994), narrative on polio in the United States had come to resonate with the Cold War mentality that pervaded public life. Disease was likened to the enemy within and the failure to act for the good of others was a betrayal of good citizenship.

This collective dedication to good public health was short-lived. By the 1980s and the HIV pandemic, according to Martin, publics were expected to see themselves as socially and economically differentiated, at risk individuals able to adapt to rapid economic and social changes. Exemplifying but complicating this shift to risk individualism, the "Grim Reaper" media campaign in Australia (Lupton 1994) and the United Kingdom's "Iceberg/Tombstone" campaign (Miller and Williams 1998) sent dual messages, since they asked all to recognize themselves at risk of HIV, but also highlighted that sex between men and injecting drug use were risk factors. This approach had the effect of deepening for some the notion that HIV was a disease of the "other" and, as it has been argued, extended forms of stigma and prejudice (Persson and Newman 2008). The communications conducted for the 2009 pandemic therefore came into this media history, an observation that did not escape some participants in the research we conducted in the United Kingdom and Australia.

Unlike some other infectious diseases, however, pandemic influenza lacks a community of interest. It pertains to all but also those who, under a pandemic gaze, are deemed vulnerable. It is a health problem that is intensely episodic and therefore lacks the strident community mobilization of chronic diseases, in the manner, for example, in which HIV affected communities have mobilized themselves to take action (Watney 2000). It is therefore difficult to sustain a conceptualization of public health—community dialectic for pandemic influenza since a pandemic is potentially about everyone and no-one in particular but also addresses the vulnerable who are seen as in need of protection and therefore passive (Stephenson et al. 2014). In contrast, Steven Epstein's history of HIV science and treatment activism showed how the incorporation of the interests of affected communities into the HIV scientific agenda helped to mobilize resources, alter modes of research governance, and support the participation of affected people in clinical trials (Epstein 1996). Epstein has also argued, however, that the dialogue is not wholly emancipatory since forms of privilege—education, class, gender, race—advantage some affected populations in their negotiations with science and government (2000, 2003), an effect that Epstein has traced into medical research more generally (2007). Paul Rabinow made a similar argument with regard to genetics research (1999), showing how different interests—across groups affected by illness and in search of cure, science, government, private capital, and media—assembled, broke, and reassembled alliances to further research for effective treatment for diseases such as diabetes. These assemblages of action on health express biological citizenship (Petryna 2003, Rose 2007), that is, claims on the right to material and symbolic resources with regard to health figured around a common biomedical identity, such as HIV or genetic illness. Such "citizenship projects" (Rose 2007, page 439) are seen to be consistent with contemporary liberal democracy. In chapter 6 we explore what turned out to be the partial, compromised pandemic citizenship of people with lung disease and part of ongoing social support and, to some extent, people with HIV, particularly in connection with what they saw as the disregard of the healthy majority for those with specific vulnerability.

Public health messages are also in a recursive relationship with popular culture and circulated in an increasingly diverse media landscape. As Wald has shown (2008), narratives on contagious, life-threatening microbes travel across the genres of science fiction, science fact, zombie horror, and alien invasion and into public health communications. In one turning of pandemic narrative, Max Brooks has written books on how to survive a zombie apocalypse (2003). Borrowing, it seems, from Brooks, the CDC in the United States created a tongue-in-cheek "zombie preparedness" program available online (CDC 2015), which traded on the popularity of the genre of zombie horror to garner the attention of publics less easy to reach with other methods (Nasiruddin et al. 2013). Writing on the zombification of popular culture and the efforts of public health, Gerlach and Hamilton have made the argument that we now live in an inescapable and proliferating "pandemic culture" (2014, online source). For instance, "viral media" social marketing approaches used to address antimicrobial resistance attempt to influence the complex ways in which media consumers use websites, social media, and the twittersphere (see, for example, @saveantibiotics; @AntibioticResis; @AMRForce) and therefore how they, too, shape the public representation of microbial threat (Wathen, Wyatt, and Harris 2008). News media stories relay public health messages on microbial threats, but also recontextualize and, potentially, overwhelm them. Addressing this complexity and in acknowledgment of the axiomatic role news and other media play in convening the public sphere and its publics (Madianou 2009), public health institutions use their own press offices to stage press releases and media conferences in an effort to shape the representation of pandemics in the interests of ruly public responses. Hallin and Briggs make the point that pandemic communications are subject to "pre-mediatization" (2015, page 96), which means that public health institutions carefully organize how pandemics and their own actions are presented to their publics.

Narrative Persuasion

Pandemic narratives, however, are not only a means of knowing: they are also seen as ways to intervene in the lives and health prospects of individuals and publics facing microbial threats. For example, narratively oriented communications on vaccination are said to improve on more traditional, information-giving approaches (Prati, Pietrantoni, and Zani 2011,

Cunningham and Boom 2013). Narrative approaches to health communication (Green 2006) and science communication more generally (Norris et al. 2005, Dahlstrom 2014) have been typified as advances on didactic methods, since they communicate affect, demonstrate cause and effect, and gesture toward the moral and ethical consequences of inaction. The use of narrative in this way is understood to "persuade otherwise resistant audiences" (Dahlstrom 2014, page 13617). An example of the turn to narrative in science edutainment is *The E-Bug Detective Game* (Farrell et al. 2011), which was designed to teach school-aged children about infection and hygiene. In this online game, the player interacts with avatars and searches for scientific evidence in places like kitchens, bathrooms, gyms, and airports to solve the puzzle of the source of an infection. Knowledge of microbes, hygiene, and infection and the related science of microbiology is conveyed in storylines with plots, characterization, demonstration of cause and effect, and attribution of responsibility. In another example, a BBC 4 radio drama *My Life with Flu* was based on a collaboration of a writer and a public health expert and featured the impact of the 1968 influenza pandemic on the lives of characters in the story (BBC Radio 4 2014). The series was conceptualized as an explicit mix of fact and fiction and indeed the drama was said to have obtained some force through scientific realism. According to Briggs (2011), in the 1990s President Bill Clinton was given a quasi-fictionalized, quasi-factual account of a bioterror event involving a genetically engineered virus to help him understand the ramifications of biological warfare in global society. Clinton, so persuaded, is said to have then enabled US government action on bioterrorism. Pandemic and related narratives, then, are not only educational assemblages of storied imagining and expert knowledge, they are thought to have political effects in the lives of individuals and nations.

The notion that narratives can persuade audiences is, however, open to some critique. There is debate in the literature whether emotive stories of the negative effects of failing to vaccinate, for example, might be counterproductive (Nyhan et al. 2014). Narrative persuasion is not far removed from the hypodermic model of communications and its address to the reasoning of the atomized, psychological individual (Young and Pieterson 2015). Narrative persuasion also glosses over the important insight that narratives can be styled and read in ways that may oppose public health. Moreover, the creation and interpretation of narratives can create opportunities for the negotiation and contestation of meaning (Ricoeur 1981), with implications for public health communications. For example, Lindy Wilbraham has explored the educational properties of *Love Lines*, a serialized program of advice on parenting in the context of South Africa's HIV epidemic, which appeared in *Fairlady*, a national women's magazine (2010). Wilbraham used one of these texts in parent groups to encourage reflection on parenting, sexuality, and gender, revealing the ways in which audiences generated their own stories in response to the *Love Lines* texts. Her analysis revealed polysemic readings and the appropriation and resistance of Western norms and knowledge on parenting and sexuality. This book, then, is partly a critical account of how expert knowledge systems of pandemic communications have appropriated narrative and how these texts are read by publics.

These uses of pandemic narrative—to educate publics, to informatively entertain radio audiences, to influence presidents, no less, and the zombification of pandemic preparedness—underline the productive dialogue of narrative, government, and science and, therefore, narrative as a mode of biopolitics. Michel Foucault's notion of biopower hinged on the realization that life was a question of politics, understood in the broad sense of the production of governable individuals and populations and the optimization of the capacities, generativity and harmony of societies (Foucault 1976). The circulation of stories on pandemics across science and into popular culture can be regarded as biopolitical action, that is, the continual and renewing examination of microbial threats, how they can be addressed and with what consequences for life.

However, the biopolitical significance of pandemic narrative reaches further than the mediation of knowledge applied to the shaping of action into the production of knowledge itself. It can be assumed, as in the examples discussed, that narrative is a means by which expert knowledge is communicated to audiences for governmental purposes. A parallel view would be that narrative helps to construct both how we are governed and the knowledge by which we are governed (Lyotard 1984). Building on this point of view, Briggs and Nichter make the case for "biocommunicability" (2009, page 189) to refer to the biopolitical rationalities that come into being at the intersection of public life, media, and the peril of contagious diseases and other threats to life. For them, social inquiry on biocommunicability attempts to:

> make sense of what factors and actors shape the ongoing production of knowledge about epidemics, how dominant and competing accounts circulate and interact, how people access and interpret information available from different sources, and what they do with it—this includes all

constituencies, from ordinary citizens to politicians and policymakers. (2009, page 197)

Alongside this focus on knowledge assemblages are questions of ethics. For Wald, the assumptions and habits of thought, othering, and stereotypes that are sustained and reworked in pandemic narratives need to be interrogated, digested, and understood to mitigate negative, and promote positive, effects:

> analysis of how the conventions of the outbreak narrative shape attitudes toward disease emergence and social transformation can lead to more effective, just, and compassionate responses both to a changing world and to the problems of global health and human welfare. (2008, page 3)

In this line of argument, pandemic tales are important modes of biomedicalizing power (Clarke 2014) that raise vital questions of individual autonomy in matters of health and medicine. Paul Farmer (1999) has argued that in the cases of tuberculosis and HIV in Haiti, long-standing dynamics of poverty, lack of investment in healthcare, and access to the benefits of biomedicine shape the healthcare options of infected people, furthering these infections and contributing to multi-drug-resistant tuberculosis. Charles Briggs and Clara Mantini-Briggs's (2003) account of a 1992 cholera outbreak in Venezuela showed how lack of investment in healthcare for the indigenous people of the Delta Amacuro region contributed to the outbreak among them and the death of some 500 people from a disease that was preventable and treatable. The 2014 outbreak of Ebola in west Africa can be understood as a reflection of structural violence produced at the intersection of a failed response to the outbreak, poorly resourced public health systems, and "misleading assumptions and myths" (Wilkinson and Leach 2014, page 137). A similar argument has been made in relation to the spread of Zika virus in 2016 and how that particular infection had worse effects for those with fewer resources (Singer 2016). Pandemic influenza, too, can be seen as revealing and deepening inequalities connected with the ways in which affluent nations of the global North spent money to protect their own citizens when health disadvantages persist in the global South and how a narrative of the other as source of contagion sustains this state of affairs (Sparke and Anguelov 2012). Pandemic influenza is commonly seen as egalitarian, predicated on the scale of the 1918–1919 pandemic, which is said to have led to the deaths of some 50 million people. But medical histories and retrospective epidemiological research of the impact of that pandemic reveal that class and access to resources shaped who got ill and how well they fared during the pandemic (Jones 2006, Mamelund 2006). Taking these lessons from other infectious diseases and the history of pandemic influenza, in this book we explore narratives on pandemic influenza as a matter of the formation of identities and the constitutive dimensions of power and, relatedly, social action on the infection. We consider how publics make themselves subject to various aspects of communications on pandemic influenza and how some of them take on the position of "at risk" while others appeared to let this identity possibility pass them by with the air of observers of a geographically, socially, and experientially distant health problem.

Pandemic Futures

Pandemic narratives, then, organize and transmit knowledge and therefore address publics as biopolitical subjects. They are said to exceed interpellation through their capacity to persuade, though, as we argue, narrative can also allow for creative appropriations and resistances. Pandemic narratives can be thought of as ramified regimes of truth with constitutive effects in science, public culture, and their hybrids, and they are also the basis for ethical debate on how societies and individuals can respond to a global threat to life. Pandemic narratives are also oriented to possible futures, a feature that helps explain why they are retold so often. Sheldon Ungar makes the point that news media from the United States, Canada, and the United Kingdom on Ebola (1998) and avian influenza (2008) show a common phasic structure: alert for members of the general public, followed by scientific deliberation and explanation about the biological particularities, effects, and risks of the pathogen and reassuring messages that the contagion is being contained. These storylines are repeated, however, not only because pandemics come and go, but because each occurrence has a future to be imagined. Pandemic narratives are captivating, in part, because, despite a generally accepted episodal structure, it cannot be known ahead of time how events will play out. The common pandemic narrative is always in tension with a pandemic as it happens. This feature of pandemic narratives helps to make them good stories, as noted, since what might happen gives the pandemic story potency. Science fiction/horror accounts of pandemic scourges are perhaps the limit case of speculation on pandemic futures. But imaginative speculation on the future of a pandemic can also be prosaic. Cameron, introduced in chapter 1, gave an account of how he had responded to the pandemic alert in 2009, indicating how he considered possible pandemic futures and then dismissed them, only to find that he had more than likely been infected. Even in the face of skepticism, or perhaps more so because of that, pandemic futures make for engaging storytelling in public and everyday life.

Importantly, speculation on pandemic futures is not only a feature of science fiction or personal experience, but also visible in the public policy focus on preparedness (Abeysinghe and White 2011, Davis, Stephenson, and Flowers 2011, Garoon and Duggan 2008). As we noted in the previous chapter, both the United Kingdom and Australia had developed their first national pandemic response plans (United Kingdom Department of Health 2007, Australian Department of Health and Ageing 2008), just before the pandemic of 2009. Both these policies made reference to preparedness as a way of managing the future, for example:

> The pandemic threat and the UK's level of preparedness are constantly evolving and this framework is a living document that will be reviewed and updated regularly. (United Kingdom Department of Health 2007, page 7)

> The overarching aim of pandemic preparedness across all sectors is to protect Australians and to reduce the impact of a pandemic on social function and the economy. (Australian Department of Health and Ageing 2008, page 2)

Preparedness plans like those from Australia and the United Kingdom share the assumption of a possible time-limited outbreak that we have seen in Cameron's story, that is, the emergence, spread, and recession of an infectious disease. Preparedness then is a bureaucratic expression of the more general speculation on what might happen in time of pandemic.

Speculation on the future is not only linked with how a future pandemic event might occur in time; it is also inevitably tied to recollection of the past (Andrews 2014), a feature of narrative imagining that was relevant to the global response to the 2009 event. It is commonly argued that there have been two other major pandemics in the previous one hundred years involving the H1N1 virus. One was the so-called Spanish influenza pandemic of 1918–1919, which supplies the benchmark for what a pandemic can do and is often referenced in public policy documents on pandemic preparedness (Australian Department of Health and Ageing 2008, Department of Health United Kingdom 2007). It is estimated that 2.5% of those infected in 1918–1919 died (Taubenberger and Morens 2006), which is a high case fatality rate for an influenza pandemic and is thought to have translated into the death of as many as 50 million people, as noted. The scale of this event is used to justify pandemic preparedness and underlines how the past shapes action in the present oriented to the management of the future, for example:

> Although little information is available on earlier pandemics, the three that occurred in the 20th century are well documented. The worst (often referred to as "Spanish flu") occurred in 1918/19. It caused serious illness, an estimated 20–40 million deaths worldwide (with peak mortality rates in people aged 20–45) and major disruption. Some residual health problems attributed to it lasted for many years thereafter. Whilst the pandemics in 1957 and 1968 (often referred to as "Asian" and "Hong Kong flu" respectively) were much less severe, they also caused significant illness levels—mainly in the young and the elderly—and an estimated 1–44 million deaths between them. (Department of Health United Kingdom 2007, page 19)
>
> In terms of the loss of human lives, the Spanish flu was unprecedented in modern times. More people died during the pandemic than were killed in the first World War. The illness came on suddenly and progressed rapidly to respiratory failure and in some instances death. Many people died from bacterial disease after infection with influenza (known as secondary bacterial infection). (Australian Department of Health and Ageing 2008, page 15)

Another, more recent, less devastating pandemic of H1N1 is also significant in narrative imagining on pandemic futures, adding some nuance to preparations for the future and foregrounding the importance of how pandemic threats are represented for publics. In 1976, an H1N1 virus outbreak was detected in the United States. At that time, the United States government sought to vaccinate the United States population to protect them from what appeared to be a severe viral infection that was thought to be a variant of the virus which led to the 1918–1919 pandemic. Unfortunately, the vaccine was linked with serious side effects, including Guillain-Barré syndrome (Dieleman et al. 2011), and there was a media controversy over the ways in which the outbreak was managed (Fineberg 2008). These events introduced risks in addition to the possible effects of an emerging infectious disease. Avoiding and managing the risk of criticism for mismanagement of a pandemic event is also a focus for public health experts, underlining the points we made earlier with regard to the "pre-mediatization" of pandemic communications (Hallin and Briggs 2015, page 96). Richard Neustadt and Harvey Fineberg cowrote an account of the 1976 outbreak in a book titled *The Epidemic That Never Was* (1983). This book title resonates quite strongly with the point we have made about the narrative tension that arises between imagining what might happen and what actually does. It also gestures toward what can be taken to be the folk-tale undercurrents of narrative on pandemic events.

Goldilocks and Other Folk-Tale Effects

Pandemic narratives, then, proliferate and travel in part because they invite imaginative speculation on what the future might bring. Implied in this consideration of pandemic futures is an emphasis on what action can be taken in the present to mitigate the possible effects of a severe infection, as in the example of preparedness policy. This consideration of the future effects of present action raises inevitable questions of moral conduct in relation to the threat to life (Freeman 2010). As we will see, many of the people who participated in our interviews and focus groups addressed themselves to just this question: How should I act now in case the pandemic is a threat to life? It is no surprise, then, to find that narrative on pandemics have a more or less implicit folkloric qualities that capture and problematize the moral implications of human agency.

The importance of folklore in pandemic narratives has been referenced by Briggs and Nichter (2009) in terms of the Goldilocks story and its underlying pedagogy of the "just right" harmonization of self-gratification with self-care under conditions of threat. Recall that in the children's story, Goldilocks seeks out experiences that are "just right" (not too big nor too little; not too hot nor too cold, not too hard nor too soft) in a situation that is ultimately dangerous when she is discovered by the bear family in their home. In their analysis of pandemics as biocommunicable events and preparedness in particular, Briggs and Nichter show how public communications are shaped to produce the most advantageous mixture of motivation and reassurance of individuals and publics. In this view, public health communications are constructed so that they encourage action on threat but without inspiring panic. This approach requires explanation of dangers for which individuals need to adopt a mode of readiness, but also calming messages that moderate unhelpful anxiety and overreaction. Like Goldilock's quest for pleasures, pandemic threat communications need to be "just right." For 2009, the just right approach translated into the "be alert, not alarmed" message that was employed across world media. Briggs and Nichter (2009) made reference to Barack Obama's April 27, 2009, speech at the annual meeting of the National Academy of Sciences, when he said: "We are closely monitoring the emerging cases of swine flu in the United States. And this is obviously a cause for concern and requires a heightened state of alert. But it's not a cause for alarm" (Obama 2009). In this and other examples, we can see that the Goldilocks framing of action supplies a readily understandable way of conveying a potentially contradictory message, that is, be ready for danger, but do not overreact. This message artfully captures the self-management of emotion (fear) and reason (readiness) required to effectively communicate with publics likely to be affected by the pandemic, a communications approach we consider in chapter 3.

Folk tales also supply a system of blame and moral status that is employed and reworked across pandemic storylines. As Wald has shown (2008), popular culture narratives on pandemic events feature characterizations of innocence, heroism, and culpability, for example, the story of Typhoid Mary in early twentieth-century New York City. In their framing of narrative and the H1N1 pandemic, Wagner-Egger et al. (2011) drew on Propp's scheme of hero, victim, and villain to explore the *dramatis personae* of the pandemic narrative in interviews with members of the general public in Switzerland in 2009. Wagner-Egger et al. make the argument that news media were seen by participants in their research as the "villain" of the pandemic narrative, whereas the medical expert emerged as "hero." This viewpoint implied that pandemic narratives have in them explicit and implicit characters whose actions and fates give meaning to pandemic storylines. As we consider in chapter 8, a particular folk tale—The boy who cried wolf—marked some of the challenges produced by the 2009 pandemic and for the public health address to individuals and populations.

Importantly too, pandemic narratives often exploit two recognizable and biopolitically significant metaphors: contagion and immunity. Both these terms signify key biomedical concepts for pandemics, but both are simultaneously and archly political. They both, therefore, do important work in circulating biopower and imbuing pandemic narratives with biopolitical force. As Wald has argued (2008), "contagion" has only relatively recently been used to denote the circulation of dangerous microbes. Previous to its modern, biomedical usage, "contagion" referred to the circulation of ideas, including and perhaps especially socially dangerous ones. Narratives on pandemic threats, then, have social revolution, upheaval, and transformation coded within them. As several authors have argued, twenty-first-century pandemics are imbued with the politics of securing the social order (Caduff 2012, Collier and Lakoff 2015, Collier, Lakoff, and Rabinow 2004, Lakoff 2008, Stephenson and Jamieson 2009). Stephenson and Jamieson (2009), for example, in their analysis of Australian news reporting on the threat of pandemic influenza and avian influenza (H5N1), show how preparedness for national emergency framed news and public policy discourse. The messages of security and preparedness that give pandemic influenza its communicative force can be read to reveal current modes of governmental address to publics and perhaps specifically post 9/11 politics (Cooper 2006). Chapter 4 explores the operation of contagion metaphors in the lived experience of our research participants. Similarly, immunity is a juridico-political concept of civil society (Cohen 2009, Esposito 2011), which has provided biomedical researchers a metaphor to capture the important sociopolitical dimensions of immunology. As we will see in chapter 5, immunity figured in the narratives of people in our interviews and focus groups, indicating the hidden and not so hidden biopolitical aspects of pandemic influenza preparedness and response.

Sarah's Epiphany

Pandemic narratives, then, are thought to have effects in public and individual life, among them to make pandemics knowable as collective and individual threat. Tales of pandemic futures are offered to publics to make them aware of what to do in the present in case of possible dangers in the future. Affective and moral pedagogies are sustained in narratives to shape subjective life and promote desirable forms of pandemic citizenship. But, then, how do individuals make sense of these stories and make use of them? In the previous chapter we considered Cameron's infection story as an example of how the pandemic was experienced by him and to highlight the themes of this book. Sarah, introduced at the beginning of this chapter, adds an important element to our developing argument due to the acute way in which the reality of the pandemic and its personal salience was made knowable for her. Sarah, along with Cameron, underlines the importance of pandemic narratives to the transformation of self-understanding and the conditioning of action on threat to life.

Sarah was a woman living in Glasgow and pregnant at the time of the pandemic in 2009. She provided an account that foregrounded the moment of coming to know herself to be an "at risk" pandemic subject, in the context of her media engagements and the meanings she found there. As noted previously, Sarah commented that she encountered the idea of herself as a member of a vulnerable group through news media:

INTERVIEWER: And how did you know that pregnant women were a vulnerable group?

SARAH: I probably saw it on the news, read it in the papers, heard it on the radio, it kind of felt everywhere. I think as well, ehm, I don't know if you were aware but there was a lady who was pregnant in [local hospital] who was really ill. You know she was on that machine for breathing and I think that it was definitely on the local news every night for weeks. And so that was just like, "Oh God, that could be me!" So I think that really struck a chord you know because she was pregnant and she was really ill. (Glasgow, 30s, Pregnant in 2009)

This account positioned news media as an important element of Sarah's experience of the pandemic and, further, as the means by which she came to recognize herself as at risk. The news that someone who was pregnant like her was unwell appeared to have been particularly important. Later in her interview, Sarah reflected again on her first experience of the pandemic:

INTERVIEWER: Can you tell me, try and remember, the first time that you heard about it.

SARAH: Ehm (pause) it was probably on the news, I imagine. I can't remember. It would either be a daily paper, or on the news. I can picture the telly, you know, the news.

INTERVIEWER: Can you remember what you saw?

SARAH: Would it be like people in China or something like that with masks on? Or when the World Health Organization first announced it was a pandemic? I can picture you know the woman in [local hospital] as well you know that kind of image obviously stays. I can picture the advertising. Was it was a guy in a lift, with the tissue?

INTERVIEWER: What did you think of that?

SARAH: "Catch it. Bin it. Kill it." or something, is that what it was?
INTERVIEWER: Yeah!
SARAH: It's obviously effective! . . . So initially, yes, I think it was just on the telly and it was, it just seemed to be every day it just seemed to be going up a level and up a level. And, you know, for me I suppose the fear was just building and building with it, thinking, "Oh God, what's going to happen? You know is everybody going to, is it going to be real?" I don't know. I think as well people were talking about the fact that it wasn't affecting over 60s the same way kind of seasonal flu would, so they were likening it to an outbreak when they were exposed to it, is that right? And they would have immunity to it or something, so it felt kind of as if they were talking about previous pandemics as well, I can vaguely remember that.
INTERVIEWER: And how did you feel about that?
SARAH: I don't know! Well every day I went round here I survived it so! I remember on one hand thinking, (sarcastically) "It's the flu . . . we'll be fine." On the other hand, you're hearing it's a pandemic and you're pregnant and you're in an at risk group and you're going to get immunized. I suppose I probably did have quite a struggle with it, you know, whether to get immunized or not.

Sarah appeared to recall the United Kingdom's "Catch it. Bin it. Kill it." advertising, underlining, like Cameron, the importance of media and health communications for her awareness and knowledge of the 2009 influenza pandemic. Her account also captured a self-questioning orientation to these messages, suggesting that understanding herself as at risk was both gradual and subject to some critical reflection. Her statement, " . . . that could be me" marked a media-related epiphany and therefore the significance of media experiences in the shaping of subjective experience (Seale 2002).

Sarah's account suggests some other effects of pandemic storytelling. When she said, "Is it going to be real?," Sarah asked of herself, "Will this affect me?," that is, "Will it come into my life?" This question echoed Cameron's infection story, discussed in chapter 1, where he was bemused and then intrigued to think that a hyped, mediated pandemic had entered his social world and body. "Is it going to be real?," then, signaled a profound question to do with the corporeality of the pandemic experience. It was also suggestive of the extensive, fictional narrative on pandemics and implied that deciding between the real and fictional is required of publics addressed by public communications and news stories. Sarah's account hinted at lingering doubt regarding the reality of the pandemic, since in its mediated form it was subject to media practices, such as hype, the assumption of which raised a question of the pandemic's realness for Sarah and others in our research. This view that the pandemic was in the media and therefore virtual is not necessarily an attempt by our research participants to engage with debates regarding the media and society relation. As we noted, we assume, as do many in this field, that media are entangled with social worlds (Kember and Zylinska 2015). We take the view that our research participants are using the idea of "the real" in opposition to the "virtual/mediated" to express the transformation of their biomedical identities, in the case of Sarah, from observer to recognizing that the pandemic narrative particular to 2009 concerned her, and for Cameron, the prospect of having been infected by H1N1. The "real" of these tales is therefore the epiphany of self-recognition and bodily transformation.

In the next chapter, we build on Sarah's epiphany of self-recognition and other dimensions of pandemic tales to explore how other people in our research engaged with the prevalent "be alert, not alarmed" message circulated by during the 2009 pandemic by public health systems and news media in the United Kingdom and Australia. On this basis, we begin to explore more fully how people in our research narrated their experiences of the 2009 pandemic.

References

Abeysinghe, S, and K White. 2011. "The avian influenza pandemic: Discourses of risk, contagion and preparation in Australia." *Health, Risk & Society* 13 (4):311–326.

Alibek, K, and S Handelman. 1999. *Biohazard: The chilling true story of the largest covert biological weapons program in the world—told from inside by the man who ran it.* New York: Delta.

Andrews, M. 2014. *Narrative imagination and everyday life, explorations in narrative psychology.* New York: Oxford University Press.

Australian Department of Health and Ageing. 2008. *Australian health management plan for pandemic influenza: Important information for all Australians.* Canberra: Australian Government, Department of Health and Ageing.

Australian Government Department of Health and Ageing. 2011. *Review of Australia's health sector response to pandemic (H1N1) 2009: Lessons identified.* Canberra: Commonwealth of Australia.

Baehr, P. 2005. "Social extremity, communities of fate, and the sociology of SARS." *Archives of European Sociology* 46 (2):179–211.

BBC Radio 4. 2014. *My life with flu.* Accessed May 1, 2017. https://www.youtube.com/watch?v=nPwwPaoEAz4

Belling, C. 2009. "Overwhelming the medium: Fiction and the trauma of pandemic influenza in 1918." *Literature & Medicine* 28 (1):55–81.

Bourdain, A. 2001. *Typhoid Mary: An urban historical*. New York: Bloomsbury.
Briggs, C. 2011. "Communicating biosecurity." *Medical Anthropology* 30 (1):6–29. doi: 10.1080/01459740.2010.531066.
Briggs, C, and C Mantini-Briggs. 2003. *Stories in the time of cholera: Racial profiling during a medical nightmare*. Berkeley: University of California Press.
Briggs, C, and M Nichter. 2009. "Biocommunicability and the biopolitics of pandemic threats." *Medical Anthropology* 28 (3):189–198.
Brockmeier, J. 2011. "Language, experience, and the "traumatic gap": How to talk about 9/11." In *Health, illness and culture: Broken narratives*, edited by L Hyden and J Brockmeier, 16–35. NewYork: Routledge.
Brooks, M. 2003. *The zombie survival guide: Complete protection from the living dead*. New York: Random House.
Caduff, C. 2012. "The semiotics of security: Infectious disease research and the biopolitics of informational bodies in the United States." *Cultural Anthropology* 27 (2):333–357. doi: 10.1111/j.1548-1360.2012.01146.x.
Camus, A. 1991 [1948]. *The plague*. New York: Vintage International.
CDC. 2014. "Pandemic influenza storybook." Accessed May 1, 2017. https://www.cdc.gov/publications/panflu/index.html.
CDC. 2015. "Zombie preparedness." Accessed May 1, 2017. http://www.cdc.gov/phpr/zombies.htm.
Charon, R. 2006. *Narrative medicine: Honoring the stories of illness*. New York: Oxford University Press.
Clarke, AE. 2014. "Biomedicalization." In *The Wiley Blackwell encyclopedia of health, illness, behavior, and society*, edited by William Cockerham, Robert Dingwall, and Stella Quah, 137–142. New Jersey: John Wiley & Sons.
Cohen, E. 2009. *A body worth defending: Immunity, biopolitics and the apotheosis of the modern body*. Durham and London: Duke University Press.
Collier, S, and A Lakoff. 2015. "Vital systems security: Reflexive biopolitics and the government of emergency." *Theory, Culture & Society* 32 (2):19–51.
Collier, S, A Lakoff, and P Rabinow. 2004. "Biosecurity: Toward an anthropology of the contemporary." *Anthropology Today* 20 (5):3–7.
Cooper, M. 2006. "Pre-empting emergence: The biological turn in the war on terror." *Theory, Culture & Society* 23 (4):113–135. doi: 10.1177/0263276406065121.
Cunningham, R, and J Boom. 2013. "Telling stories of vaccine-preventable diseases: Why it works." *South Dakota Medical Association, Sioux Falls*. Special Edition:21–26.
Dahlstrom, M. 2014. "Using narratives and storytelling to communicate science with non-expert audiences." *Proceedings of the National Academy of Sciences* 111 (Supplement 4):13614–13620.
Darabont, F. 2010. *The walking dead*. United States, New York: AMC Studios.
Davis, M, N Stephenson, and P Flowers. 2011. "Compliant, complacent or panicked? Investigating the problematisation of the Australian general public in pandemic influenza control." *Social Science & Medicine* 72 (6):912–918.
Department of Health United Kingdom. 2007. *Pandemic flu: A national framework for responding to an influenza pandemic*. London: Author.
Dieleman, J, S Romio, K Johansen, D Weibel, J Bonhoeffer, M Sturkenboom, and VAESCO-GBS Case-Control Study Group. 2011. "Guillain-Barré syndrome and adjuvanted pandemic influenza A (H1N1) 2009 vaccine: Multinational case-control study in Europe." *BMJ* 343:d3908.

Epstein, S, ed. 1996. *Impure science: AIDS, activism and the politics of knowledge.* Berkeley: University of California Press.
Epstein, S. 2000. "Whose identities, which differences? Activism and the changing terrain of biomedicalisation." Paper presented at HIV and Related Diseases Conference (HARD) Social Research Conference, Gazebo Hotel, Sydney, May 13, 2000.
Epstein, S. 2003. "Sexualising governance and medicalising identities: The emergence of 'state-centred' LGBT health politics in the United States." *Sexualities* 6 (2):131–171.
Epstein, S. 2007. *Inclusion: The politics of difference in medical research.* Chicago: Chicago University Press.
Esposito, R. 2011. *Immunitas: The protection and negation of life.* Cambridge: Polity.
Farmer, P. 1999. *Infections and inequalities: The modern plagues.* Berkeley: University of California Press.
Farrell, D, P Kostkova, J Weinberg, L Lazareck, D Weerasinghe, D Lecky, and C McNulty. 2011. "Computer games to teach hygiene: An evaluation of the e-Bug junior game." *Journal of Antimicrobial Chemotherapy* 66 (Supplement 5):v39–v44.
Fenn, E. 2001. *Pox Americana: The great smallpox epidemic of 1775–82.* New York: Hill and Wang.
Fineberg, H. 2008. "Preparing for avian influenza: Lessons from the 'Swine Flu Affair.'" *Journal of Infectious Diseases* 197 (Suppl 1):S14–S18.
Foucault, M. 1976. *The birth of the clinic: An archaeology of medical perception.* London: Tavistock Publications.
Frank, A. 1995. *The wounded storyteller: Body, illness and ethics.* Chicago: University of Chicago Press.
Freeman, M. 2010. *Hindsight: The promise and peril of looking backward.* Oxford: Oxford University Press.
Galarce, E, S Ramanadhan, and K Viswanath. 2011. "Health information seeking." In *The Routledge handbook of health communication, second edition*, edited by T Thompson, R Parrot, and J Nussbaum, 167–180. New York: Routledge.
Garoon, J, and P Duggan. 2008. "Discourses of disease, discourses of disadvantage: A critical analysis of National Pandemic Influenza Preparedness Plans." *Social Science & Medicine* 67 (7):1133–1142. doi: 10.1016/j.socscimed.2008.06.020.
Gerlach, N, and S Hamilton. 2014. "Trafficking in the zombie: The CDC zombie apocalypse campaign, diseaseability and pandemic culture." *Refractory: A Journal of Entertainment Media* June 24, Electronic source: http://refractory.unimelb.edu.au/2014/06/26/cdc-zombie-apocalypse-gerlach-hamilton/
Green, M. 2006. "Narratives and cancer communication." *Journal of Communication* 56 (s1):S163–S183. doi: 10.1111/j.1460-2466.2006.00288.x.
Greenhalgh, T. 2006. *What seems to be the trouble? Stories in illness and healthcare.* Oxford: Radcliffe Publishing.
Hallin, DC, and CL Briggs. 2015. "Transcending the medical/media opposition in research on news coverage of health and medicine." *Media, Culture & Society* 37 (1):85–100. doi: 10.1177/0163443714549090.
Hilton, S, and K Hunt. 2011. "UK newspapers' representation of the 2009–10 outbreak of swine flu: One health scare not over-hyped by the media?" *Journal of Epidemiology and Community Health* 65:941–946.
Hilton, S, and E Smith. 2010. "Public views of the UK media and government reaction to the 2009 swine flu pandemic." *BMC Public Health* 10:697.

Hine, D. 2010. *The 2009 influenza pandemic: An independent review of the UK response to the 2009 influenza pandemic*. London: Pandemic Flu Response Review Team, Cabinet Office.
Holland, K, and W Blood. 2012. "Public responses and reflexivity during the Swine flu pandemic in Australia." *Journalism Studies* 14 (4):523–538. iFirst: doi:10.1080/1461670X.2012.744552.
Honigsbaum, M. 2013. "Regulating the 1918-19 Pandemic: Flu, stoicism and the Northcliffe Press." *Medical History* 57 (2):165–185. doi: http://dx.doi.org/10.1017/mdh.2012.101.
Jones, E. 2006. "Politicizing the laboring body: Working families, death, and burial in Winnipeg's influenza epidemic, 1918–1919." *Labor* 3 (3):57–75. doi: 10.1215/15476715-2006-005.
Kember, S, and J Zylinska. 2015. *Life after new media: Mediation as a vital process*. Cambridge, MA: MIT Press.
Kleinman, A. 1988. *The illness narratives: Suffering, healing and the human condition*. New York: Basic Books.
Kolata, G. 1999. *Flu: The story of the great influenza pandemic of 1918 and the search for the virus that caused it*. New York: Touchstone.
Lakoff, A. 2008. "The generic biothreat, or, how we became unprepared." *Cultural Anthropology* 23 (3):399–428.
Lupton, D. 1994. *Moral threats and dangerous desires: AIDS in the news media*. London: Taylor & Francis.
Lyotard, J. 1984. *The postmodern condition: A report on knowledge*. Minneapolis: University of Minnesota Press.
MacPhail, T. 2014. *The viral network: A pathography of the H1N1 influenza pandemic*. Ithaca: Cornell University Press.
Madianou, M. 2009. "Audience reception and news in everyday life." In *The handbook of journalism studies*, edited by K Wahl-Jorgensen and T Hanitzsch, 325–337. Abingdon: Routledge.
Mairal, G. 2011. "The history and the narrative of risk in the media." *Health, Risk & Society* 13 (1):65–79.
Mamelund, S. 2006. "A socially neutral disease? Individual social class, household wealth and mortality from Spanish influenza in two socially contrasting parishes in Kristiania 1918–19." *Social Science & Medicine* 62 (4):923–940.
Martin, E. 1994. *Flexible bodies: Tracking immunity in American culture from the days of polio to the age of AIDS*. Boston: Beacon Press.
Miller, D, and K Williams. 1998. "The AIDS Public Education Campaign, 1986–90." In *The circuit of mass communication: Media strategies, representation and audience reception in the AIDS crisis*, edited by D Miller, J Kitzinger, K Williams, and P Beharrell, 13–45. London: Sage.
Nasiruddin, M, M Halabi, A Dao, K Chen, and B Brown. 2013. "Zombies—A pop culture resource for public health awareness." *Emerging Infectious Diseases* 19:809+.
Neustadt, R, and H Fineberg. 1983. *The epidemic that never was: Policy-making and the swine flu scare*. New York: Vintage.
Norris, S, S Guilbert, M Smith, S Hakimelahi, and L Phillips. 2005. "A theoretical framework for narrative explanation in science." *Science Education* 89 (4):535–563. doi: 10.1002/sce.20063.

Nyhan, B, J Reifler, S Richey, and G Freed. 2014. "Effective messages in vaccine promotion: A randomized trial." *Pediatrics* 133 (4):e835–e842.

Obama, B. 2009. Remarks by the President at the National Academy of Sciences Annual Meeting, April 27, 2009, https://www.whitehouse.gov/the-press-office/remarks-president-national-academy-sciences-annual-meeting, accessed October 25, 2015.

Oshinsky, D. 2005. *Polio: An American story*. New York: Oxford University Press.

Persson, A, and C Newman. 2008. "Making monsters: Heterosexuality, crime and race in recent Western media coverage of HIV." *Sociology of Health & Illness* 30 (4):632–646.

Petersen, A, M Davis, S Fraser, and J Lindsay. 2010. "Healthy living and citizenship: An overview." *Critical Public Health* 20 (4):391–400.

Petryna, A. 2003. *Life exposed: Biological citizens after Chernobyl*. Princeton: Princeton University Press.

Prati, G, L Pietrantoni, and B Zani. 2011. "Influenza vaccination: The persuasiveness of messages among people aged 65 years and older." *Health Communication* 27 (5):413–420. doi: 10.1080/10410236.2011.606523.

Rabinow, P. 1999. *French DNA: Trouble in purgatory*. Chicago: University of Chicago Press.

Ricoeur, P. 1981. *Hermeneutics and the human sciences: Essays on language, action and interpretation*. Cambridge: Cambridge University Press.

Rose, N. 2007. *The politics of life itself: Biomedicine, power and subjectivity in the twenty-first century*. Princeton: Princeton University Press.

Seale, C. 2002. *Media and health*. London: Sage.

Seale, C. 2003. "Health and media: An overview." *Sociology of Health and Illness* 25 (6):513–531.

Sharf, B, L Harter, J Yamasaki, and P Haidet. 2011. "Narrative turns epic: Continuing developments in health narrative scholarship." In *The Routledge Handbook of Health Communication*, edited by T. Thompson, R Parrott, and J. Nussbaum. New York: Routledge.

Singer, M. 2016. "The spread of Zika and the potential for global arbovirus syndemics." *Global Public Health* 12 (1):1–18. doi: 10.1080/17441692.2016.1225112.

Soderbergh, S. 2011. *Contagion*. United States: Warner Bros. Pictures.

Sparke, M, and D Anguelov. 2012. "H1N1, globalization and the epidemiology of inequality." *Health & Place* 18 (4):726–736. doi: http://dx.doi.org/10.1016/j.healthplace.2011.09.001.

Squire, C. 2007. *HIV in South Africa: Talking about the big thing*. London: Routledge.

Stephenson, N, M Davis, P Flowers, E Waller, and C MacGregor. 2014. "Mobilising 'vulnerability' in the public health response to pandemic influenza." *Social Science & Medicine* 102:10–17.

Stephenson, N, and M Jamieson. 2009. "Securitising health: Australian newspaper coverage of pandemic influenza." *Sociology of Health & Illness* 31 (4):525–539.

Taubenberger, J, and D Morens. 2006. "1918 Influenza: The mother of all pandemics." *Emerging Infectious Diseases* 12 (1):15–22.

Ungar, S. 1998. "Hot crises and media reassurance: A comparison of emerging disease and Ebola Zaire." *British Journal of Sociology* 49 (1):36–56.

Ungar, S. 2000. "Knowledge, ignorance and the popular culture: Climate change versus the ozone hole." *Public Understanding of Science* 9:297–312.

Ungar, Sheldon. 2008. "Global Bird Flu Communication: Hot Crisis and Media Reassurance." *Science Communication* 29 (4):472–497.

United Kingdom Department of Health. 2007. *Pandemic flu: A national framework for responding to an influenza pandemic*. London: Author.

Wagner-Egger, P, A Bangerter, I Gilles, E Green, D Rigaud, F Krings, C Staerklé, and A Clémence. 2011. "Lay perceptions of collectives at the outbreak of the H1N1 epidemic: Heroes, villains and victims." *Public Understanding of Science* 20 (4):461–476. doi: 10.1177/0963662510393605.

Wald, P. 2008. *Contagious: Cultures, carriers, and the outbreak narrative*. Durham: Duke University Press.

Warner, M. 2002. *Publics and counterpublics*. Cambridge, MA: Zone Books.

Wathen, N, S Wyatt, and R Harris, eds. 2008. *Mediating health information: The go-betweens in a changing socio-technical landscape*. Houndmills: Palgrave Macmillan.

Watney, S. 2000. *Imagine hope: AIDS and gay identity*. London: Routledge.

Wells, HG. 2005 [1898]. *The war of the worlds*. London: Penguin.

Wilbraham, L. 2010. "Parental communication with children about sex in the HIV/AIDS epidemic in South Africa: Cultural appropriations of Western parenting expertise." In *HIV treatment and prevention technologies in international perspective*, edited by M Davis and C Squire, 87–108. Houndmills: Palgrave Macmillan.

Wilkinson, A, and M Leach. 2014. "Briefing: Ebola—myths, realities, and structural violence." *African Affairs* 114 (454):136–148.

Williams, G. 2013. *Paralysed with fear: The STORY OF POLIO*. Houndmills: Palgrave Macmillan.

Young, L, and W Pieterson. 2015. "Strategic communication in a networked world: Integrating network communication theories in the context of government and citizen communication." In *The Routledge handbook of strategic communication*, edited by D Holtzhausen and A Zerfass, 93–112. Abingdon: Routledge.

3
"Be Alert, Not Alarmed!"

> I did feel there was a conscious effort to try not to panic people. If you see what I mean? So how do you get people to kind of get a sense of urgency without panicking? (laughs) You know. I definitely got an idea of both of those things. (Rebecca, Glasgow, 30s, Pregnant in 2009)

As this quotation from Rebecca's interview indicated, and as we noted in the previous chapter, communications on the pandemic strived to establish "a sense of urgency without panicking" people. This important message pervaded official communications and news media. For example, on April 27, 2009, two days after the World Health Organization (WHO) announced a "public health emergency of international concern" (2011), the *Geelong Advertiser*, a regional newspaper in the Australian state of Victoria, carried an article titled "Be alert for swine flu but no need to panic." In the article, Australia's then–chief medical officer, Jim Bishop, was quoted saying, "We don't think we should be very worried at the moment. . . . We're in a good state of preparedness" (Jenkins 2009). This early news story, then, made a link between the "Be alert, not alarmed" message and the preparedness and response orientation of the public health system. This message was repeated in the media in the first few days of the "emergency." Bishop was also quoted in the *Sydney Morning Herald* on April 27, saying, "We should be aware but I'm not overly alarmed at this point" (AFP, Robotham and Pearlman et al. 2009). The United Kingdom's chief medical officer, Liam Donaldson, was quoted in *The Guardian* on May 1, saying he was "concerned, but not alarmed" at the news that the WHO had declared a Phase Five pandemic (Bowcott et al. 2009). The telling and retelling of "Be alert, not alarmed" showed how preparedness rationality was transferred into communicative action with affected populations. This message, occurring as it did so early in the news media on the pandemic, is suggestive of "pre-mediatization" (Hallin and

Pandemics, Publics, and Narrative. Mark Davis and Davina Lohm, Oxford University Press (2020).
© Oxford University Press.
DOI: 10.1093/oso/9780190683764.001.0001

Briggs 2015, page 96), the situation where messages from the WHO and national governments emanated from communications plans that prefigured how best to set the narrative emphases in the news and therefore how publics were to be most advantageously addressed. Holland and Blood (2012) have commented that the journalists they interviewed regarding news stories on pandemic influenza were focused on establishing the message "Be alert, not alarmed." As we noted, Briggs and Nichter (2009) have argued that the "Be alert, not alarmed" message was a key communications theme in 2009 and was expressed most ably in speeches made by President Obama. In Canada, news media audiences were asked to "stay vigilant" and to not panic (CBC News 2009).

These preparedness messages asked publics to temper overreaction (alarm and panic) with vigilance and readiness to act (be alert). This modulation of affect by reason and the associated poising of publics in readiness was the idealized citizenship of pandemic preparedness and response. It represented the active cultivation of a pandemic subject attuned to efforts to manage a global emergency that involved a high degree of uncertainty. "Be alert, not alarmed" was also a subjective position that echoed previous epochs where pestilence and war coincided, as we discussed in chapter 2 in relation to the campaigns on polio and Cold War politics in the United States and in the case of the 1918–1919 pandemic, World War I, and the imperative defense of nation.

This "Be alert, not alarmed" messaging has been deployed more recently. In 2016 during the news media interest in Zika virus, the *chef de mission* of the Australian Olympic team noted: "We don't want to scare our potential team members, but I suppose it's a case of 'alert but not alarmed' " (Channel Seven News 2016). In another television news item, the journalist called on their health editor to comment on the risk of Zika. The health editor reported that Australia's chief health officer had said: "We are wary of it. We are alert to it but it is not something we should be panicking about just yet" (Channel Seven News 2016). These "Be alert, not alarmed" messages indicate that, in general, public authorities are invested in an ideal pandemic citizen, ready to act and not complacent, but also not so worried as to be likely to overreact.

As discussed, Briggs and Nichter (2009) have referred to this government of public affect and reason as the "Goldilocks" approach to communication on the H1N1 virus, since it sought out a "just right" message that expressed urgency without stimulating unhelpful panic. Rebecca suggested the "just right" message in her quotation from the beginning of this chapter. If we can assume that this Goldilocks message was "pre-mediatized" in preparedness and response plans or elsewhere, the emphasis placed on facts in the media releases of the public health system marked an appeal to reason and therefore an effort to close off speculative, inflammatory discourse. This appeal to reason may also be seen as apposite given that researchers have argued that publics now express risk fatigue, that is, publics have been bombarded with messages of impending risks and have therefore become exhausted by, or inured to, them (Joffe 2011). A calming message of readiness may therefore be seen as more sustainable than a raised level of anxiety. Folkloric communication, or more particularly, the preparedness message of "Be alert, not alarmed" is, in this view, a biopolitical technology in its own right.

In this chapter, we consider the biopolitical resonances and implications of the "Be alert, not alarmed" message. We focus on the interview and focus group talk that examined what it meant to be asked to get ready for a public health emergency and therefore how members of the general public engaged with the communicative biopolitics of the 2009 pandemic. The perspectives developed in this chapter are important for understanding how preparedness rationality is translated into communicative action and how this message was received, interpreted, appropriated, and, at times, resisted.

Public Communications on the 2009 Pandemic

As we noted in the previous chapter, during the 2009 pandemic, public health communications were articulated through public service and news media. According to the United Kingdom's review of the management of the pandemic (Hine 2010), public communications commenced in late April with a United Kingdom–wide information campaign on television, radio, print media, and a booklet delivered to every household. This media activity featured the "sneezing man" and "Catch it. Bin it. Kill it." images and messages. The booklet contained this instruction: "As the situation changes, you should keep up to date by watching TV, listening to the radio, checking the internet and looking out for announcements in the press." Posters were present in National Health Service (NHS) buildings and workplaces, and advice was seen on bus shelters, billboards, and shopping trolleys. The National Pandemic Flu Service—a web-supported telephone service modeled on NHS Direct—was commenced in England on July 23, and similar services came online, soon after, in Scotland, Wales, and Northern Ireland. According to the United Kingdom review, 2.7 million people in England used the National Pandemic Flu Service. On August 13, it was publicly announced in the United Kingdom that some members of the community were at heightened risk, including pregnant women and people with specific respiratory and immune system vulnerabilities. Daily media briefings were held by governments across the United Kingdom from the end of April into early July, and epidemiological updates were made available on a weekly basis. In Scotland, the deputy first minister and the cabinet secretary for health and well-being conducted media briefings and appeared on television. Tailored communications were developed for pregnant women and for people attending the Hajj during the later months of 2009.

In Australia, the Commonwealth Government organized a national media campaign on television, radio, and print media in four phases (Australian Government Department of Health and Ageing 2011). Phase 1 (May 2009) advised the general public on the hygiene and social distancing methods that could be used to moderate the transmission of the virus. These strategies included covering the mouth and nose when sneezing or coughing, washing hands and using hand sanitizers, keeping all surfaces clean, avoiding the sharing of personal items, and avoiding close contact with others. Information was disseminated at this time regarding the heightened risk for those in vulnerable groups. Phase 2 (September 2009) alerted the population to the availability of the H1N1 vaccine and was followed by Phase 3 (December 2009), which provided information on the vaccine for children. Phase 4 (March 2010) addressed the apparent misconceptions held by the general public regarding the H1N1 vaccine. A parallel communications strategy was developed for indigenous communities. As in the United Kingdom, a health emergency website was established for both the public and professionals. Updated on a daily basis, the website provided epidemiological information and advice on prevention and treatment. According to the Australian Government review, 28 million hits were recorded on the website for the period between May 2009 and September 2010. Telephone hotlines were also used in Australia, and the Commonwealth Government addressed the news media through briefings, including 50 or so press conferences chaired by the chief medical officer and/or the Commonwealth Government health minister.

Similar activity was undertaken in Australian States and Territories. In Victoria and New South Wales (NSW), Departments of Health established their own incidence rooms and surveillance mechanisms and managed contact tracing and clinical services. Each state developed Internet-based resources for professionals and the general public. Chief health officers in both states liaised with the Commonwealth and conducted press conferences. For example, a news item titled "The Swine Flu—Are We Ready?" (Miller et al. 2009) was written by the health correspondent of *The Age*—Melbourne's serious broadsheet newspaper—on May 2, in the days after the public health emergency was announced. The item reflected on preparedness, previous pandemics, and the work of the WHO on the outbreak in Mexico. It featured short quotations from the Commonwealth health minister and Victorian chief health officer. In response to a question regarding the hoarding of food in the case of a severe pandemic, the health minister was quoted saying, "There are in some cases people panicking unnecessarily. I want to reassure people that there currently are no confirmed cases of swine flu in Australia." The chief health officer was quoted saying, "Australians react extremely well in situations of crisis, whether it be a bushfire or flood."

In general, our research participants had retained only some recollection of public health communications, perhaps not surprisingly since the interviews were conducted between two and three years after the peak of the pandemic in Australia and the United Kingdom. Mary, in her 30s, lived in Glasgow and was pregnant during the pandemic. She recalled some of the communications used in 2009, including the self-triage telephone services and the United Kingdom's "Catch it. Bin it. Kill it." campaign, but not clearly, and with some coaching from the interviewer. Mary first commented on the messages that asked people to use the telephone services rather than present at the doctor's surgery, a procedure she said may have been flawed:

INTERVIEWER: What did you think of the kind of media coverage and the kind of the NHS coverage?
MARY: I was quite surprised actually by the NHS coverage more than anything because I thought, I hadn't really seen it in previous years and I thought they're being quite purposeful about the communication that they're giving flu this year. They're being very purposeful and it's being a bit different than what I'd seen in the past and maybe it is actually the same but we hadn't heard about it. When I think about it, if [Mary's daughter] was sick today I'd be saying, "[Mary's daughter], get yourself an appointment and get straight down that doctor and see what he can see." But I kind of knew that wasn't what you were meant to do this time. You weren't supposed to go down to your doctor and you weren't meant

to do that and I thought, "Well that's kind of different from normal." But, you know, maybe it is for flu just the same but I didn't know it because it wasn't as publicized before. Ehm . . . you know I thought, "Well you're not supposed to do that, you're supposed to call NHS 24 and you're supposed to speak to somebody rather than go down there," which makes sense but then I think "Well, how can you diagnose somebody over the phone about that?" It's kind of . . . I don't know, I don't know whether I trust that phone diagnosis system. (Glasgow, 30s, Pregnant in 2009)

Mary's account showed awareness that individuals were asked to use the Internet and telephone services in preference to attending doctor's surgeries. Her account signaled that this new mode of engagement was something of a disruption to her normal practices and that the notion of telephone-based diagnosis was met with some mistrust. Like many other of the United Kingdom respondents, Mary's narrative also drew in some skeptical reference to the NHS. Washer and Joffe, in their research on hospital-acquired infections in the United Kingdom, have made note of what has been referred to as "NHS-bashing," a common narrative in news media and in the accounts of those people they interviewed (Washer and Joffe 2006). Our UK interviews did not denigrate the NHS, overtly, but they did repeatedly cast doubt on it as a public institution, as Mary did in her account. Australians in our research did not criticize public health services in this way, perhaps because healthcare delivery is run by state and local organizations. Mary went on to discuss the advertising used in the United Kingdom, in a playful banter with the interviewer:

INTERVIEWER: And do you remember the kind of ads on the TV?
MARY: Was that the ones with people sneezing and touching things?
INTERVIEWER: Yeah, tell me more about what you do remember about that.
MARY: Like touching hand rails and things like that. Is that the one you mean? Where they were like on a bus and they would leave like a kind of trail where they were going. Is that the one yeah?
INTERVIEWER: Whichever ones you remember!
MARY: I don't know if that's some kind of Vick's Vapour Rub advert or whether that's like a swine flu advert which is probably a really bad sign for swine flu adverts not being very memorable. (laughs) That's the only thing I can take from it that nobody remembers the swine flu advert.
INTERVIEWER: And they kind of blur with the commercial products.

MARY: Yeah. They need to do a better job of medicalizing their NHS advertising. Yeah. Well that's one I thought of and it probably isn't, I don't think it was a commercial one, though, I think it was an NHS one, but I just don't remember if that was a swine flu one or whether it was a general one. But I don't think they do general flu ones, so maybe it was swine flu. But the one I'm thinking of, the guy went out and was coughing and sneezing all over the place and touching things as he went and there was a big push on hand washing and, you know, that kind of thing, and it couldn't have been commercial because I would've remembered the product itself.
INTERVIEWER: And what was the—
MARY: —And it was kind of the bin it . . . oh I can't remember—
INTERVIEWER: Go on, say it! (laughs) Say it. What do you reckon it is?
MARY: "Catch it something bin it," I can't remember—
INTERVIEWER: You almost said it.
MARY: Catch it, something, bin it, something like that. "Catch it. Kill it. Bin it." That was it, yeah. Yeah they had some kind of advert.
INTERVIEWER: The guy in the lift? Do you remember that?
MARY: I don't know if I remember that—
INTERVIEWER: He's in a lift and he (makes the noise of a sneeze). Anyway, I've been looking at the ads so I've got a better record.
MARY: And was there one on public transport I seem to remember most? Where the guy was like touching things on places and other people were as well. I think actually maybe that sticks, because, I think "Yeah, that could happen" (laughs) "That could happen to me."

The interviewer referred to the well-known television advertisement that featured a man sneezing in a lift, exposing his companions to his infection (NHS 2009). Mary, however, may have referred to advertisements on public transport that used still images to send a similar message (Hine 2010). This account usefully demonstrated that audiences were exposed to and recalled different aspects of the pandemic communications. Australian participants reinforced this perspective that communications and media engagements were multiple and depended on the life circumstances of the individual. Lara, a Sydney-sider in her 30s with lung disease, commented that television was her main form of engagement with the pandemic message. Despite Lara's elevated risk status and as someone who attended hospital and her doctor regularly to manage her lung disease, media and reflections on the media were integral to her experience of the pandemic:

INTERVIEWER: Did anyone close to you have any personal encounter with the swine flu?
LARA: No, no. We just saw the stuff on TV. I don't know anyone that got sick from it personally.
INTERVIEWER: I guess, you know, there's lots of kind of media comments about it, wasn't there?
LARA: Yeah, there was heaps on TV. There were a couple of warning pamphlets at the hospital. But I don't think they took any extra, you know, or they didn't appear to take any extra precautions or, you know, anything with it.
INTERVIEWER: Can you remember if there were any posters and that up?
LARA: Yep, we definitely saw literature up at the hospital. And our GP he's pretty relaxed with stuff like that. He's like, "It's more media hype than, than actual illness," you know, "Don't worry about it." Which is fine, but definitely the hospital had stuff up and, you know, literature that you could take home about it. (Sydney, 30s, Lung disease)

Like Mary from Glasgow, Lara was addressed by several media forms, including television news reports and posters in her hospital. Importantly, Lara commented that her doctor had advised her to not overreact to the messages in the media, echoing comments made by Cameron, as discussed in chapter 1. In chapter 7, we discuss this idea of "media hype" in connection with other research. Lara also nominated media as her main form of experience of the pandemic in response to the question, "Did anyone close to you have any personal encounter with the swine flu?" Lara's negative response, and others like it from the interviews and focus groups, indicated that the 2009 pandemic was highly mediated; it was experienced largely—for some even wholly—through news and other media, a perspective that underlines the importance of media narratives for pandemic experience.

Critical Awareness

Our research participants made reference to the preparedness message and engaged with the idea of "be alert, not alarmed," but in ways that showed critical awareness. They were able to recognize the preparedness message and discuss it as a communication strategy of public health systems in the United Kingdom and Australia and/or an effect of the news media. Opinions varied with regard to what the message was for, how it was executed, and how it should be digested and enacted. This talk on being alert to the possible meanings and implications of "Be alert, not alarmed" was reflected in the critical stance our research participants afforded themselves in their narratives of being reluctantly or cautiously persuaded into "at risk" subjectivity, or otherwise, as the pandemic emerged in their social worlds. What follows implies that further refinement of the preparedness message and how to deliver it may not be as important for public health as acknowledgment of, and working with, the critical skills audiences bring to their engagements with public health communications and news media.

Lara, introduced earlier, recalled the preparedness message. Picking up on the idea that the news media had hyped the pandemic story, however, she commented that it appeared not to have been easy to stage the message to best effect:

INTERVIEWER: What about the government responsibilities? What do you think those are? How did the government respond at that time?
LARA: I think there was too much fear portrayed in the press. And yes, it was lethal, but the people who were dying were very young or very old and sick, to my knowledge. And it has to be taken seriously but—
INTERVIEWER: So you think maybe the media trivialized it a wee bit?
LARA: Exactly, exactly. Perhaps the message was lost through all the fear campaign and, you know, what was it that was said, "Be aware, not alarmed." You know? (Sydney, 30s, Lung disease)

Lara's comment indicated that communicating on the pandemic was difficult because some were severely affected but not all, which is in itself a complicated message to give to the general public. Lara therefore touched on the everyone/vulnerable people duality we raised in chapter 2. Pandemic communications address the population and ask them all to take care, but also identify that some are vulnerable. This dual message may get lost, particularly in the context of what is seen to be news media hype, even if the actual content of the news is factual. The idea that media hype might overwhelm the more subtle messages of pandemic preparedness reiterates the primacy of media as social form as opposed to the meanings it conveys in its content and reveals the constitutive power of the general framing provided by the well-known and culturally elaborated pandemic narrative.

The tension noted by Lara with regard to the tendency of media hype to overwrite the preparedness message was taken up in Rebecca's interview. The quotation from Rebecca was presented at the beginning of the chapter as an example of our research participants' critical engagement with the preparedness message. The quotation gathers additional meaning, however, in the context of the discussion that preceded it of Rebecca's deliberations on the H1N1 vaccine. Vaccination was a concern for Rebecca since, as a pregnant woman, she was in a priority group according to the United Kingdom's approach. She said that the pandemic message in connection with the vaccine and more generally was taken by her to be an address to the balance of reason and emotion circulated widely in news media:

> I felt the main message, if you like, that I was getting was that the vaccine is safe and the risks associated with the vaccine are less than the risks associated with the infection. That was what I took from it as the main things. But at the same time as that there was a sort of sense of urgency that, "We really would like everyone to be vaccinated please because we think that if this were to be a major outbreak that it would be a disaster." At the same time as that sense of urgency there was also a sense of trying to quieten things down and giving you enough information to let you know it was quite serious, but by also tailoring it with the, "But those people were already ill" comment at the end. So there was kind of two levels, because on the one hand they obviously wanted everyone to be vaccinated or at least they wanted everyone in these groups to be vaccinated and they obviously felt it's really important to be vaccinated, as they do every year with the flu jab, you know, they're always trying to get people to have the flu jab every year. But at the same time I did feel there was a conscious effort to try not to panic people. If you see what I mean? So how do you get people to kind of get a sense of urgency without panicking? (laughs) you know. I definitely got an idea of both of those things. And it did seem to be on the radio, generally I don't tend to watch the news on the television as much, I tend to always listen to the news on the radio, and I definitely seem to remember there was a story about swine flu on the radio all the time. Like every bulletin had a story about it. Like they were definitely trying to infiltrate everybody's daily thinking about it, yeah. (Glasgow, 30s, Pregnant in 2009)

Rebecca showed awareness of the potential contradiction between motivating people to take action in tandem with efforts to calm them down and like Lara, the ambiguities of the dual message that everyone/the vulnerable should take care. This dual message is seated in biomedical knowledge, but, given Lara and Rebecca's comments, has the effect of undermining itself since the statement of vulnerability implies that actually not everyone need worry too much. In this view, facts work against themselves and undermine the preparedness message, an effect that can be traced into the action of biomedicine's own knowledge systems on itself (Clarke and Shim 2011). Rebecca also very ably identified what could be called "panic titration"; the cultivation of just enough emotional energy to mobilize precautionary behavior but without provoking unhelpful overreaction, as we discuss in the next section. Her talk on the preparedness message and its links into the decision to vaccinate underlined the point we made at the beginning of this chapter that "Be alert, not alarmed" can be thought of as a biopolitical technology of pandemic affect.

Rebecca's discussion of preparedness and vaccines also mobilized the authority of public health in the repeated use of "they." In this extract, the interviewer probed Rebecca's prior reference to a generic "they" in relation to the pandemic threat message:

INTERVIEWER: When you say "they" you said "they were very keen" and "they kept telling us?"
REBECCA: Yeah.
INTERVIEWER: Who are "they?"
REBECCA: (laughs) (pause) Well whenever it was on the news. The news would always tell you all the ins and outs and I suppose they're being fed by the public health department and they want to make sure that everyone knows it's not just random people who are dying. It's people who are unwell that this is affecting badly. I suppose it's a mixture of the media and government health bodies.
INTERVIEWER: And you said, "They seemed to be very careful."
REBECCA: Yeah, they were. I always felt like it was an attempt to not have a mass panic. It's not completely normal, healthy people who have got flu and then suddenly they die. It's people who have underlying health problems and they're already at a lowered level of health anyway and that's why the virus affects them particularly badly. And I did feel that every time I heard anything, or anything on the news I remember specifically

thinking, it was any time you heard about it you could practically predict that it was the last line of the story would be " . . . and this person had underlying health difficulties" you know, like all the time. So I suppose I kind of took it to be that they're trying to encourage people to be, you know, it's not just an indiscriminate killer! (laughs) You know, it's affecting these people because they're already of a kind of weakened immune system.
INTERVIEWER: And there's a sense of someone being quite deliberate?
REBECCA: Oh yeah definitely! Yeah, managing panic. Yeah definitely, definitely it's a kind of public health body who are in charge of that, I don't know. I haven't really thought about who "they" are before! (laughs)

Demonstrating critical awareness of not only the pandemic message but its production for the general public, Rebecca made reference to the public health communications–media nexus and the transparent styling of messages to avoid panic. Rebecca's phrase, "managing panic," signaled her awareness that the pandemic message addressed emotions. Rebecca's and other accounts like it also showed that the pandemic message was understood by a knowing public already able to detect and critique how they were being advised during the emergency and in particular that they recognized that the news media stories on the pandemic were populated by "characters" and in particular the voice of the public health expert. Moreover, Rebecca spoke of public health experts as actively shaping the knowledge presented in news stories. Public communication was not then simply a matter of the transmission of information for publics to absorb. Individuals appear to be able to decode how expert knowledge is woven into news media and other modes of communication of the preparedness message. Accounts like Rebecca's pervaded our interviews and focus groups and could be taken to constitute some support for the manner in which communications and media were managed during the 2009 pandemic since participants demonstrated that they had comprehended the advice and made assumptions that it carried with it the authority of public health systems. The accounts also show, however, the high degree of message decoding of which publics are capable, applied to the content of the texts but also the politics surrounding how they are assembled.

Dave, a man in his 60s living in Glasgow and with no reported health problems, also referred to "they" as the public health experts of communications and news media. His account exhibited recognition of the imperatives and risks of blame faced by the "they" of pandemic government:

INTERVIEWER: And now where did you get all your information from?
DAVE: Just the newspapers.
INTERVIEWER: Just newspapers?
DAVE: Aye, newspapers and occasionally there was programmes on the telly or sections in the news that said, you know, "This is the problem that's going to happen," and so forth and that they felt that it could be . . . At the end of the day if people don't think of these things and something goes wrong they get blamed and then they get criticized when they do shout about it and nothing happens. So I suppose they're walking a path that's very difficult, eh, to please everybody and at the end of the day you're better to prepare for what may be. (Glasgow, 60s, No disclosed health problems)

The uncertainties of pandemic influenza surfaced in Dave's rather sympathetic account of the challenges that were faced by the public health system in the United Kingdom. The conundrum Dave referred to—that experts could be criticized for not acting if the pandemic turned out to be serious, but also criticized for acting if nothing in the end happened—is consistent with the official UK review of the public health system's management of the 2009 pandemic (Hine 2010). These accounts carefully explained that in the throes of a deeply uncertain emerging pandemic a precautionary approach was justified, a position that Dave, remarkably enough, appeared to endorse. The important point of Dave's account though was that it demonstrated in another way the reflexive manner in which publics appeared to have engaged with the "Be alert, not alarmed" message.

Marlene, who was in her 30s and lived in Sydney, also revealed herself to be hyper-aware of the preparedness message, perhaps because she had lung disease. But Marlene said that authorities appeared to have stifled panic, and counterproductively so:

I think . . . telling people not to panic . . . well for me it . . . I remember those kind of news reports at the time. I remember being a bit upset about it 'cause I thought like I really want people to take it seriously. I'm not sure exactly what part of the pandemic that report was from, whether it was at the start or near the end. I really did want people to take it seriously and I think if they're worried about it, I think they were justified in feeling worried about it. And I think telling people not to panic sort of made it, like trivialized it a little bit and made it seem as though it wasn't maybe as trivial as what it, what it was for me. I guess yeah, I didn't really like that kind of reporting 'cause panic's probably not a good thing but it's better than being blasé about it, I guess. (Sydney, 30s, Lung disease)

Marlene appeared to have been speaking from her position as someone more affected by the threat of the pandemic than others, given the risk implied by her health status. For her, "Be alert, not alarmed" had underplayed dangers, though she also acknowledged that panicky messages might have been counterproductive. Her account implied that Marlene felt separated out from others, as interpellated in the negative since for her the pandemic was potentially more serious than the calming voice of public health expertise seemed to have implied. Her account underlined the critical awareness that publics appeared to have brought to their reception of the preparedness message. It reiterated how a universalizing message—"Be alert, not alarmed"—could divide publics in terms of their relative vulnerability to the threat posed by a public health emergency (Stephenson et al. 2014). Marlene's account, in particular, pointed to the ways in which the preparedness message articulated with the social and biomedical situation of members of the general public, a perspective that we explore in chapter 6.

Panic Titration

Lara, Rebecca, Dave, and Marlene, like others in our research, in various ways, engaged with how the "Be alert, not alarmed" message could be used to greatest effect. They all recognized the political import of the message and understood also that the reasoned containment of ungovernable emotion was key. Marlene, argued that, while overreaction was not wanted, too much emphasis on calming the population may undermine the preparedness project. These different positions on how to achieve the Goldilocks message (Briggs and Nichter 2009)—the just right combination of reason and emotion—is an approach to governmentality that resonates with the "vigilant and ready" society or "metastable" society, as Massumi has argued in relation to the war on terror (2009). In Massumi's view, publics are suspended in a state of alertness, ready to act if need be, but on an ongoing basis, such that preparedness becomes a governmental and subjective norm. Penelope Ironstone-Catterall has written of pandemic risk governmentality grounded in the modulation of anxiety, or "neurotic citizenship" as she called it (2011, page 91). Writing on preparedness for a possible H5N1 pandemic, Ironstone-Catterall argued that the possibility of a future pandemic crisis is not simply a field of calculative reason, it also inspires anxiety that gives risk its meaning and motive force and therefore is the background on which publics are addressed. This view inflects the risk society thesis with the meaning of "state of anxiety" wherein an anxious public is necessary to contemporary politics and government. In related research with public health professionals involved in the management of the response to the 2009 pandemic (Davis, Flowers, and Stephenson 2013, Davis 2017), this Goldilocks problem emerged in an interview:

PUBLIC HEALTH PROFESSIONAL: Well, there was a lot of advice coming out for them [publics] and it was a fine balance getting the right message. Now, they [authorities] were basically saying, "This is a serious disease. We are doing all these things. Most people are fine but you still have to be cautious," kind of thing. So a kind of message of reassurance but tempered with a sort of precautionary approach, "Watch and be careful. But it was all under control." And I think they [the public] bought into that quite well, and were reassured for the most part. I didn't get any flavor of panic other than initially the odd person a bit flustered when they heard that they'd got the swine flu.

MD: When you say panic?

PUBLIC HEALTH PROFESSIONAL: I think when you're planning there was a lot of consideration of whether, what measures could be taken to make sure there wasn't panic. I think panic was thought to be one of the consequences of having a pandemic.

MD: You actually talked about that when you were planning before swine flu?

PUBLIC HEALTH PROFESSIONAL: Yeah like bulk buying and things like that and people not wanting to go into work because they were scared or not wanting their children to go to school that kind of thing.

MD: So acting in ways that would distract the plans?

PUBLIC HEALTH PROFESSIONAL: Or just disrupt society and create more problems, you know.

[later]

MD: You said it was a fine line. Do you want to talk a bit more about that?

PUBLIC HEALTH PROFESSIONAL: I was just trying to say that, if you say everything is fine then people might become blasé and not think it's a big deal. So when the doctor says you're not meant to go to work with these symptoms, you've got swine flu, or you need to come to hospital because you're pregnant and it is going to be serious, they might not obey the instructions. But on the other hand you don't want people all being so nervous that, like I said, they start behaving oddly. So, it's just being able to get a message across . . . don't panic. You've got things to be done. You're not to panic, but you are to follow these instructions and be a responsible citizen kind of thing. (Public health professional, 2010, United Kingdom)

The finely tuned execution of the Goldilocks preparedness message and relatedly the cultivation of panic titrated just enough to mobilize publics to readiness was a preoccupation for public health, according to this interviewee. As noted previously, an ideal pandemic citizenship is implicated in the "Be alert, not alarmed" message, and it is referenced in this interview extract, too. Communicative action styled to fabricate docile citizens, able to act if called on to do so, has been a feature of the pandemic narrative for some time. As we have noted, Honigsbaum (2013), in his research on the 1918–1919 influenza pandemic, developed an argument regarding the classed stoicism detectable in newspapers and other documents in circulation at that time in Britain. Because the pandemic coincided with the final stages of World War I, it was reported in light of the war effort and, therefore, a presiding imperative to foster British courage in the face of the threat presented by Germany. Edwardian notions of class and conduct meant that the ruling elites had a duty to demonstrate stoical self-management to less well-educated classes, since it was believed that overanxious reaction to the pandemic made soldiers more likely to be infected, and infected severely, and to therefore render themselves less useful for the war effort. The 2009 pandemic's "Be alert, not alarmed," can be seen to have made a similar appeal to publics to take the position of the informed and calm and to eschew the position of the ill-informed and overanxious. There is then, perhaps, a hidden class politics in contemporary communications on pandemics. The ideal subject of the communications as they pertain to pandemics is perhaps an educated, emotionally self-regulating one. The ruling class who dutifully demonstrate and promote "Be alert, not alarmed" are no longer the landed gentry and aspirational bourgeoisie of the Edwardian period, but the cadre of professionals, government bureaucrats, and politicians who articulated the authoritative voice of public health across media in time of pandemic.

This focus on the mitigation of counterproductive anxiety can also be traced into psychological theory on health communications and behavior, but not without some contradiction, since these theories assume that motivation depends on a degree of emotional stimulation. In this frame, a key objective of communications is to motivate people to adopt new behaviors, strengthen and or redeploy existing behaviors, and suspend and or dispense with risk-producing ones (Flowers et al. 2016). The psychological theory informing these efforts relies on an assumption that proximity to a feared stimulus—in this case the threat of pandemic influenza—will motivate behavior change. This idea was pioneered by Irwin Rosenstock (1974) in connection with polio vaccination and has been elaborated and modified into frameworks of psychological responses to pandemic threats that encompass perceptions of the severity and likelihood of infection, anxiety regarding the pandemic, and belief in the efficacy of the hygiene and social isolation methods advocated by public health experts.

Emotions are complicated, too, in the sense that they are mercurial and open to displacement. Anxiety, for instance, can be expressed in many ways and sometimes in humor, which may be a cathartic release of anxiety and also exercise a kind of alternative citizenship of pandemic preparedness. Cameron's account from chapter 1 of his probable infection with the H1N1 virus was couched in humorous, self-mocking terms, marking the narrator as critical of media hype but also in the end confronted, ironically, with the virus in his own body. Similarly, some of the gay men with HIV spoke of H1N1 in a joking manner. As we explore in chapter 6, HIV-positive people in our research, though they were identified as a vulnerable group and given priority for vaccination in the United Kingdom and Australia, were focused on HIV treatment and how it would be affected by possible influenza infection. Bobby, from Glasgow and in his 40s, made this point:

INTERVIEWER: You know the interview is about swine flu? Do you remember swine flu vaccination?

BOBBY: I remember all the hype and hysteria and . . . (sighs) the media nonsense and the political stuff and all that. I remember having it. I did have it [the vaccination] yes, but I didn't ask for it, I didn't go out of my way and say "I want swine flu, I want swine flu!" At the end of the day it became a bit more of a running joke, you know, the swine flu and stuff like that. (laughs) It became more of a running joke if I remember right, people sneezing and people giggling and saying "swine flu!" (laughs). I did have the jag [vaccination], yes, I had the jag.

INTERVIEWER: Just tell me more about this idea of being a bit of a joke.

BOBBY: I think that the usual media hysteria, the governments and media they just drummed something, they've got to run with something, a newspaper has got to run with something, so the media and government throw it to the media and say, "Here go and fucking stoke up the hysteria with this nonsense, tell them how many people are going to die around the world and how we've had to buy all these vaccines and get the message out there!" So they just bombard you with nonsense, the media and stuff like that and that's what I remember about it and that's what the joke was "Oh it's another 5 people die of swine flu!" Where? Fucking Mexico or something like that "Oh it's on its way to Britain!" Aye right, give us some fucking peace. (laughs) You know and it just became a bit of a joke so that if anybody had a bit of a cough or a sneeze or anything like that at work it was just like "swine flu!" and you just made a laugh and a joke about it and you used to say, "What's the side effects of swine flu, a wee curly tail?" But it was more of a laughing stock than anything else because of the media, the media frenzy and all the hype and that nonsense around about it and that's what it was, just nonsense you know so, I wouldn't say it was a big thing, more of a laughing stock at the time.

INTERVIEWER: When you talked about the mass media hype and you talked about the government, how do you think they're all connected?

BOBBY: Oh they're all linked! The governments use newspapers, the newspapers use governments. It's a two-way thing with these lot and this stuff. If they want anything out there they just throw it to the media and that's it, they've got to get it across somehow, whether it's news, newspapers, television news, adverts and stuff, they just throw it out there and make sure it gets in around the public adverts on buses and, you know, the posters, bill boards and stuff like that everywhere. It's just it just seems to take over sometimes. In those circumstances they just bombard you with it, the information. (Glasgow, 40s, HIV positive)

Bobby caricatured the media and government response and crudely but compellingly pointed out the circuit of mutual dependence they form in the case of pandemic and beyond. His story of "swine flu" as a source of fun indicated that the emotions associated with the pandemic did not only run along the axis of calm to panic. Other more complexly relational emotions and related practices—in this instance humor and joking at work—were also implicated. Bobby, like Cameron, depicted himself as not the ideal citizen of preparedness, though it also appeared that according to him, he vaccinated when asked to do so. It is argued that gendered notions of emotional responses to illness shape how men and women account for their responses to health problems (Connell 2012). Perhaps Bobby's humor and Cameron's self-effacement articulate masculinity fitted to the pandemic threat. Gendered talk on pandemic influenza did emerge in interviews and focus groups, a feature of the research we explore in chapter 6 in connection with the biopolitical subject positions adopted by some of our research participants.

Prepared Citizens

The critical awareness that we found in interviews and focus groups and the multiple perspectives on the emotional undercurrents of the preparedness message indicated that publics were active in their pandemic engagements and creatively so. In this critical, creative engagement, respondents also laid claim to autonomy and self-regulation, figured around their identities as knowledgeable and, at times, skeptical. In this our respondents expressed citizenship-like claims on how they conducted themselves in relation to the messages on the pandemic (Petersen et al. 2010, Petryna 2003, Rose 2007), shaping themselves therefore as "preparedness citizens."

Preparedness citizenship was exercised by our participants in several ways and appeared to be a taken-for-granted assumption. Deb, from Melbourne and with a new baby in 2009, made a claim for her right to "make a judgment" with regard to how to enact preparedness:

> I think if media beefs-up something too much, it makes people blasé about things. And so you've gotta be careful with that. . . . So as long as the facts are coming through with how many cases and where then people can sort of make a judgment on how bad they think it really is. Yeah. And then that would determine how they act and whether they're gonna be a bit more, you know, cautious about it or not. (Deb, 30s, new baby in 2009)

Deb appeared to be aware of the medias' role in shaping the preparedness message and in particular the Goldilocks problem that too much hype may make people turn away from the message. Deb argued, however, that deciding what to do was up to her and people like her and therefore the presentation of factual information was the basis for the decision-making of the individual. This citizenship-like claim on autonomy implied that the public response was not necessarily shaped in a direct way or that the psychological individual can be influenced through knowledge of their beliefs and motivations. A sense on the part of public of their own right to decide appeared to mediate action. The autonomy of pandemic citizens, however, is constrained by a feature of the expert knowledge that is used to sustain the public health approach to pandemic risk. Knowing that a pandemic is afoot relies on pooling information gathered from multiple sources. This has been axiomatic to public health at least since John Snow's famous research on the source of a cholera epidemic in nineteenth-century London (Pollock 2012). In an early form of contact tracing of affected people and the collection of information regarding their daily life, Snow revealed a pattern of the spread of the disease that was not apparent to individuals or even to doctors caring for those affected by the infection. As the reviews of the 2009 pandemic showed (Australian Government Department of Health and Ageing 2011, Hine 2010, WHO 2011), public health authorities were said to have carefully followed up news reports of unusual influenza-related data in Mexico and to have examined information coming from national surveillance systems across the globe. The global view, which gives a sense of the event and scale of the outbreak, depends on networks of knowledge generation, sharing, and deliberation. Preparedness citizens depend on these systems of knowledge generation and are therefore tied into public health knowledge systems. Deb's claim to "make a judgment" is only partially an expression of autonomy, since life and its management is tied so closely to expert knowledge systems (Giddens 1990).

The assumption of autonomy, however, appeared to be important to the people who participated in our interviews and focus groups. Like Deb, Vincent, from Sydney and with no reported health problems, took a critical position on communications and media. He indicated that an ability to "read the media" was a necessary element of the effective navigation of the preparedness message:

INTERVIEWER: So you mentioned the media previously and that's kind of part of your recollection of the 2009 swine flu. In general, did you feel it was exaggerated or did you feel the media has a tendency to exaggerate the issue?

VINCENT: Yeah, I mean my, my view is the government, I don't think the government necessarily was exaggerating and I don't, I think, you know, gut instinct says that they probably did what they should have done. I don't, I think media, probably hyped it up for some people. Those people who don't know how to I s'pose read the media and understand that the media do jump on these sort of stories and will run with them. And for some people they probably were overly concerned. More concerned than they should have been. And, therefore you do get this rush. As soon as they've got a sniffle they'll rush. And that does cause problems for those who really do or really may have it. So I think my view is I'm probably more skeptical, actually, of the media than I am of the government in this. And I think the government, the media have a lot to probably answer for in creating those issues. (Sydney, 40s, No disclosed health problems)

Vincent's account echoed the critical stance of others in our research and also the classed stoicism that Honigsbaum linked with the 1918 pandemic. Vincent positioned himself as able to decode the media, unlike others without such advantages, marking himself as not the unruly, uneducated other. In addition, some of our respondents gave the impression that their ability to enact preparedness was linked with social advantages. Gill lived in inner Melbourne and was late in her pregnancy when the pandemic broke out. According to her, she came to know of the potential risks associated with H1N1 due to her husband's work in a local hospital:

They did a lot of disaster planning. He was involved in a lot of planning of what they would do if it came to Melbourne. And he came home talking about it and saying that, "If it comes to Melbourne, I don't want you catching public transport," and this, that and the other. So I guess I was very aware of it before the general public. (Melbourne, 30s, Pregnant in 2009)

Gill's story was an important reminder that for some people, news reports or public communications were not the first way in which they found out about the pandemic, though we can surmise that communicative activity on pandemic risk was being undertaken in the hospital in which her partner worked. Because of this particular feature of her life circumstances, Gill also found that the information provided by public health authorities came too late:

INTERVIEWER: So have you got any comments about the way in which you think the government handled the swine flu pandemic?

GILL: I felt like the official recommendations from the government came a bit late. Like it's hard to remember now, two and a half years later. I felt like the government was running behind me in terms of how serious it was and what precautions should be taken. I don't think they called for pregnant . . . I think later in the piece they called for pregnant women to be very careful. And perhaps to avoid public transport. That was months after I'd done it. Well, so I wasn't mad.

INTERVIEWER: So it took a while you thought for those messages to come through.

GILL: Yes it did, yes.

INTERVIEWER: I can imagine that would have been really concerning, given the fact that you were pregnant.

GILL: I think by the time the recommendations came out I had given birth and it didn't bother me.

Gill's account signaled that events in her own life coincided with the pandemic only roughly and she appeared to have taken steps to reduce her risk in advance of public communications. Her account suggested the value of time to the management of pandemic risk. Time is an important element of pandemic preparedness and response, and, as we have seen, the temporal character of pandemic as event in time informs public communications and news media. According to Gill, time in the form of forewarning appeared to have personal value and to provide the basis for a kind of enhanced, savvy, preparedness citizenship. Gill's reference to forewarning showed also how the preparedness rationality being established in the hospital where her partner worked was employed in personal life. This account of the use of the methods of preparedness and response derived from the hospital setting breaks down in another way the idea of the public as a unity and of preparedness citizenship as external to public health systems and as only an object of preparedness and response plans. In some circumstances, personal action on pandemic risk is enacted in concert with the public health system's address to its own preparedness and response. Gill's account also suggests a form of privilege gained by advanced warning from her links into the public health system, another way in which public engagement is nuanced and perhaps even stratified. In an analysis of the social impacts of HIV testing technologies that permit individuals to ascertain their HIV serostatus at home, Jonathan Banda (2015) suggests that biomedical processes are implicated in forms of social stratification of access to biomedical innovation and related health outcomes. The comments of our research participants indicate that advantages do appear to accrue among those who are networked into public health systems and therefore not wholly reliant on media and other communications.

"Be alert, not alarmed" was an important message for publics in 2009, but its overtly unifying address masked divisions and negations. The message was one way of extending the "just right" combination of alertness to danger and reasonable action and in some respects was a key political and communications achievement of the 2009 pandemic. But as we have seen, the request to all to adopt this preparedness position placed some people outside of the "alert and not alarmed" general public since they had also come to think of themselves as potentially more severely affected. Some respondents also pointed out the self-defeating nature of a message that sustained the view that there was no cause for alarm, but also that some were very threatened; or conversely, that sought to mobilize the vulnerable against threat while reassuring the general public against unreasonable panic.

These perspectives indicate that the preparedness message does not come into public life in a vacuum. Individuals bring their interpretation skills into their reception of the preparedness message, a feature of public engagement that is no doubt why the preparedness is so thoroughly premediatized by public health systems (Briggs and Nichter 2009). We argue, however, that pandemic communications cannot only be managed through the styling and repetition of "Be alert, not alarmed." Comprehension of the relational aspects of pandemic storytelling is also vital for public health—in this view, it is not so much what is said but the qualities and materialities of the relationships between public health systems and their publics. Public communications on pandemics are dialogical in only a limited sense, and there would seem to be little scope for collaborative storytelling in the way that, for example, might be possible in a face-to-face situation, such as a clinical encounter (Greenhalgh 2006) or in a research interview (Gubrium and Holstein 2008). In these contexts, the practical and ethical dimensions of life, knowledge, and expertise can be negotiated in a productive manner. In pandemic communications, dialogue and relationality are somewhat interrupted and messengers do not necessarily hear whether their message has been taken up by their audiences in a direct sense. This basic communicative challenge appears to have been taken up in public policy rationality. For example, the 2014 version of the *Australian Health Management Plan for Pandemic Influenza* referred to the need for public communications that were "two-way" and made note of the value of "listening" to publics (Australian Department of Health 2014, page 63). This approach to feedback on the transmission of information was said to depend on in vivo market research, the monitoring of social media, and a Q&A website where publics can pose questions and air their opinions (Australian Department of Health 2014, page 63). It remains to be seen how well these forms of communications feedback will work and whether they will approximate the dialogical and relational dimensions of telling and listening that operate in other domains of life. Addressing these challenges will be crucial if the turn to narrative persuasion in public health communications is to be useful and effective.

References

AFP, AAP, G Kwek, J Robotham, and J Pearlman. 2009. "Global alarm as killer swine flu spreads." *Sydney Morning Herald*, April 27. Accessed October 25, 2015. http://www.smh.com.au/world/global-alarm-as-killer-swine-flu-spreads-20090426-ajjo.html.

Australian Department of Health. 2014. *Australian health management plan for pandemic influenza*. Canberra: Commonwealth of Australia.

Australian Government Department of Health and Ageing. 2011. *Review of Australia's health sector response to pandemic (H1N1) 2009: Lessons identified*. Canberra: Commonwealth of Australia.

Banda, J. 2015. "Rapid home HIV testing: Risk and the moral imperatives of biological citizenship." *Body & Society* 21 (4):24–47.

Bowcott, O, S Carrell, I Traynor, and S Morris. 2009. "Swine flu: First case of UK human transmission suspected." *The Guardian*, May 1. Accessed October 15, 2015. http://www.theguardian.com/world/2009/may/01/swine-flu-spread-uk.

Briggs, C, and M Nichter. 2009. "Biocommunicability and the biopolitics of pandemic threats." *Medical Anthropology* 28 (3):189–198.

CBC News. 2009. "Canada 'well positioned' if pandemic alert level raised: Health officer." Accessed July 12, 2018. https://www.cbc.ca/news/canada/canada-well-positioned-if-pandemic-alert-level-raised-health-officer-1.831606.

Channel Seven News. 2016. "Virus fears." January 15, 2016.

Clarke, A, and J Shim. 2011. "Medicalization and biomedicalization revisited: Technoscience and transformations of health, illness and American medicine." In *Handbook of the sociology of health, illness, and healing: A blueprint for the 21st century*, edited by B Pescosolido, J Martin, J McLeod, and A Rogers, 173–199. New York: Springer.

Connell, R. 2012. "Gender, health and theory: Conceptualizing the issue, in local and world perspective." *Social Science & Medicine* 74 (11):1675–1683.

Davis, M. 2017. "'Is it going to be real?': Narrative and media on a pandemic." *Forum Qualitative Sozialforschung / Forum: Qualitative Social Research* 18 (1). http://nbn-resolving.de/urn:nbn:de:0114-fqs1701187.

Davis, M, P Flowers, and N Stephenson. 2013. "'We had to do what we thought was right at the time': Retrospective discourse on the 2009 H1N1 pandemic in the UK." *Sociology of Health & Illness* 36 (3):369–382.

Flowers, P, M Davis, D Lohm, E Waller, and N Stephenson. 2016. "Understanding pandemic influenza behaviour: An exploratory biopsychosocial study." *Journal of Health Psychology* 21 (5):759–769.

Giddens, A. 1990. *The consequences of modernity*. Cambridge: Polity.

Greenhalgh, T. 2006. *What seems to be the trouble? Stories in illness and healthcare*. Oxford: Radcliffe Publishing.

Gubrium, J, and J Holstein. 2008. "Narrative ethnography." In *Handbook of emergent methods*, edited by S Hesse-Biber and P Leavy, 241–264. New York: Guilford Press.

Hallin, DC, and CL Briggs. 2015. "Transcending the medical/media opposition in research on news coverage of health and medicine." *Media, Culture & Society* 37 (1):85–100. doi: 10.1177/0163443714549090.

Hine, D. 2010. *The 2009 influenza pandemic: An independent review of the UK response to the 2009 influenza pandemic*. London: Pandemic Flu Response Review Team, Cabinet Office.

Holland, K, and W Blood. 2012. "Public responses and reflexivity during the Swine flu pandemic in Australia." *Journalism Studies* 14 (4): 523–538. iFirst: doi:10.1080/1461670X.2012.744552.

Honigsbaum, M. 2013. "Regulating the 1918–19 pandemic: Flu, stoicism and the Northcliffe Press." *Medical History* 57 (2):165–185. doi: http://dx.doi.org/10.1017/mdh.2012.101.

Ironstone-Catterall, P. 2011. "Narrative the coming pandemic: Pandemic influenza, anticipatory anxiety and neurotic citizenship." In *Criticism, crisis, and contemporary narrative*, edited by P Crosthwaite, 81–94. London: Routledge.

Jenkins, M. 2009. "Be alert for swine flu but no need to panic." *Geelong Advertiser*. Accessed February 5, 2015. http://infoweb.newsbank.com.ezproxy.lib.monash.edu.au/iw-searc...tion=doc&p_docid=127D5373E77BB250&p_docnum=122&p_queryname=11.

Joffe, H. 2011. "Public apprehension of emerging infectious diseases: Are changes afoot?" *Public Understanding of Science* 20 (4):446–460.

Massumi, B. 2009. "National enterprise emergency: Steps toward an ecology of powers." *Theory, Culture & Society* 26 (6):153–185.

Miller, N, M Toy, J Medew, and Agencies. 2009. "The swine flu—Are we ready?" *The Age*. Melbourne.

NHS. 2009. "UK swine flu alert." Accessed May 1, 2017. https://www.youtube.com/watch?v=3F9W551mZy0.

Petersen, A, M Davis, S Fraser, and J Lindsay. 2010. "Healthy living and citizenship: An overview." *Critical Public Health* 20 (4):391–400.

Petryna, A 2003. *Life exposed: Biological citizens after Chernobyl*. Princeton: Princeton University Press.

Pollock, G. 2012. *An epidemiological odyssey: The evolution of communicable disease control*. Dordrecht: Springer.

Rose, N. 2007. *The politics of life itself: Biomedicine, power and subjectivity in the twenty-first century*. Princeton: Princeton University Press.

Rosenstock, I. 1974. "Historical origins of the health belief model." *Health Education Monographs* 2 (4):328–335.

Stephenson, N, M Davis, P Flowers, E Waller, and C MacGregor. 2014. "Mobilising 'vulnerability' in the public health response to pandemic influenza." *Social Science & Medicine* 102:10–17.

Washer, P, and H Joffe. 2006. "The 'hospital superbug': Social representations of MRSA." *Social Science & Medicine* 63 (8):2141–2152. doi: http://dx.doi.org/10.1016/j.socscimed.2006.05.018.

World Health Organization (WHO). 2011. *Implementation of the International Health Regulations (2005). Report of the Review Committee on the Functioning of the International Health Regulations (2005) in relation to Pandemic (H1N1) 2009. Report by the Director-General.* Geneva: World Health Organization.

4
Contagion

> I would isolate my children. Mind you, in the past I may not have isolated them for a long enough time because of those things like having to go to work and them missing out on their education. I would have to sort of gauge if I could afford to lose money by not going to work. (Brigitte, Melbourne, 40s, School-age children)

Brigitte's comment on the isolation of her children referred to the methods used to mitigate the spread of the influenza virus. More often referred to as social distancing, these "nonpharmaceutical" means of stemming transmission were used in 2009 and included asking people with confirmed infection and those in their families to self-quarantine at home; advising people with symptoms to avoid others, and; encouraging the public in general to avoid those with symptoms (Australian Government Department of Health and Ageing 2011, Hine 2010). Some schools were closed in Scotland (Health Protection Scotland 2010) and Australia (Australian Government Department of Health and Ageing 2011), but governments did not stop public transport and major sporting events. To support social distancing and also to reduce the potential for overwhelming numbers of people attending clinics and hospitals, telephone and online self-triage systems were activated in England on July 23 (Rutter et al. 2014).

Social distancing was seen as a crucial element of the public health response to the pandemic during the period of time it took to find a suitable vaccine. As we have noted previously, vaccination commenced in Australia on September 30, 2009 (Australian Government Department of Health and Ageing 2011) and in the United Kingdom on October 21 (Hine 2010), five to six months after the World Health Organization announced a public health emergency on April 25 (World Health Organization 2011). The other pharmaceutical method of pandemic mitigation—antiviral treatment (Tamiflu/oseltamivir)—was used in 2009 and continues to be a component

Pandemics, Publics, and Narrative. Mark Davis and Davina Lohm, Oxford University Press (2020).
© Oxford University Press.
DOI: 10.1093/oso/9780190683764.001.0001

of pandemic preparedness (Australian Department of Health 2014, Public Health England 2014). Antivirals, however, are thought to be most efficacious if given soon after infection (Zambon 2014), and there is currently some debate with regard to the evidence that antivirals are effective for the management of pandemic influenza (Butler 2014).

As indicated by Brigitte, however, the practical considerations of childrearing, working life, and education do appear to limit efforts to implement social distancing, as borne out in survey research conducted at the time (Mitchell et al. 2011, page S138). No one we interviewed or in a focus group reported that they had been asked by public health authorities to self-isolate, although some spoke of having known others who did this and many spoke of attempts to reduce social interaction in response to supposed infection, because of their own vulnerability, or as a general principle of influenza risk management. Along with the practicalities of establishing and sustaining social distancing, people spoke of these methods in ways that revealed them to depend on others, underlining the cooperation required to make social isolation work.

Social distancing is also framed by a contagion imaginary and the related ideas that dangers like pandemics arise elsewhere and in other people. Contagion, as Wald has explained (2008) and as we noted in chapter 2, is a key metaphor of pandemic narrative with ramified meanings that help to explain the circulation of microbial life in human populations but that also help to bring biopolitical rationalities into narrative on pandemics. Contagion has an etymology in the concept of touch and has been used to denote the circulation of ideas that constitute collective life, particularly dangerous ones like revolution (Wald 2008, page 2). As Wald has shown, biomedical science exploits the political meaning of contagion—the transmission of dangerous ideas from one person to another—to help give explanatory force to germ theory and to establish epidemiology and the discipline of infectious diseases, among other knowledge effects. The biomedical appropriation of contagion has also helped to bring biomedical knowledge into politics, making the contagion metaphor an important site for the production of biopolitical meanings. The narratives generated in our interviews and focus groups exhibit these ideas of social distance as defense against contagion and therefore mobilize ideas of delimited space and distance from others as protection from danger. Preparedness policy and the responses to the 2009 pandemic also relied on this ancient idea of enclosed space set against the incursion of microbial threat.

But the biopolitics of contagion are shown to be more than simple ideas of self defined against the dangerous other and the spatial separation afforded by social isolation from the dangerous other. Also important are networks and flows that traverse space and that explain distance differently, as we will see, and that are important to the application of biopolitical reason. A central lesson from Foucault's *Security, Territory, Population* (2007), for instance, is that security is not simply a mechanism for the protection of the population from an encroaching threat. Over time it came to be understood as the survival of individuals and populations through the flows of goods, people, and ideas, among other matters. As Foucault put it in relation to the case of the social and economic survival of the town:

> what was at issue in the eighteenth century was the question of the spatial, juridical, administrative, and economic opening up of the town: resituating the town in a space of circulation. (2007, page 13)

Conversely, the erection of boundaries and withholding of exchange can lead to the erosion of social well-being (Collier and Lakoff 2015, Lakoff 2015). Enforced social distancing was used in 2003 during the SARS outbreak in Toronto, where over 13,374 people were quarantined (Sanford and Ali 2005). Quarantine was not used for the 2003 SARS outbreak in Hong Kong, but the government did require citizens to wear facemasks (Baehr 2005). SARS was regarded as a severe infection because it was associated with a high rate of mortality: in some estimates as much as 15% of those infected, overall, and more than 50% of those infected who were aged 65 years and older (World Health Organization 2003). Toronto's citizens, for the most part, complied with the quarantine, but not without costs to themselves and the city's economy. In Hong Kong, dissenting citizens forced the government to publish online a list of SARS-affected buildings, against the prevailing wisdom of authorities. The SARS experience in Toronto and Hong Kong strained the public health–publics relationship, which as we will see in a later chapter is sustained through fragile systems of trust in expert knowledge and the action of government. Enforcing social distancing in the form of isolation and quarantine has to be carefully considered for its disruption of the connections and flows that secure political, economic, and social life.

In addition, distance proved to be a weak form of protection in the case of the 2009 pandemic. For example, the first case of H1N1 in Mexico was notified on March 17, 2009 (Centers for Disease Control and Prevention 2009).

The first case in Scotland was confirmed on April 27 (Health Protection Scotland 2010), and in Australia on May 6 (Australian Government Department of Health and Ageing 2011). While social distancing may have had value for containable infections like SARS, its utility for influenza viruses in early twenty-first-century, hyperconnected global societies is an open question and is the subject of extensive retrospective modeling research using mortality and morbidity data from 2009 (Cauchemeza et al. 2011).

Moreover, our increasingly hyperlinked, globalizing economic and cultural exchanges have altered what is meant by distance (Appadurai 2013). Globalization dynamics, for example, are said to have dissolved the link between space and time such that we no longer consider ourselves separated simply by distance (the kilometers between Glasgow and Melbourne) but in terms of the time it takes to travel distance (24 hours or so between Glasgow and Melbourne) (Cohen and Kennedy 2000, Scholte 2000). Pandemics are complexly articulated with these changing networks and rapid flows of globalization. The emerging infectious diseases narrative, in particular, implies that the transmission of influenza viruses are facilitated in part by the increased speed of travel and the numbers of people, animals, and goods that now flow across the globe (Morse 1995) and is true for other infections, such as Zika virus (Singer 2016) and antimicrobial resistant infections (UK Review on Antimicrobial Resistance 2016). In addition, then, to its practical challenges, dependence on cooperative action, and connotations of a contagion imaginary, social distance is itself a contradictory mixture of enclosure and networked flow. As we will see, the experiential narratives of our research participants showed that ideas of networked, dissolving space coexisted with, and interrupted, ideas of social distance as a method of defense against contagion.

Social distance also has a specifically narrative association in relation to alienation, or narrative distanciation as it is sometimes called (Czarniawska 2004). In chapter 3, we explored the idea that the expression of pandemic narratives in public life lack the dialogical and relational character that is possible in interactional life. We suggested that therefore, attempts made by public health systems to address and engage publics also inevitably lack the kinds of coproduction of narrative that is said to be hallmark of narrative medicine (Greenhalgh 2006) and that is axiomatic to critical approaches in narrative research on lived experiences (Andrews, Tamboukou, and Squire 2013). In addition, narrative does not always bring tellers and listeners into sympathetic or empathic connection: audiences can be made other in some narratives and turned away from stories in a negated interpellation—"not you"—of their subjective experience of public culture. It is important to recognize how narratives can be turned to the alienation of audiences, particularly as narrative persuasion is being promoted, it seems to us in a somewhat uncritical manner, as a way to influence individuals to protect themselves in our era of emerging infectious diseases.

This chapter explores, therefore, narrative on the enactment, meanings, and tensions of social distance in connection with the historical advent of the 2009 pandemic. Our interest is not simply in how people navigated social distance as a method of reducing their risk of infection, though that is relevant. Our focus is on the symbolic loading of social distance and how notions of enclosed and networked space coexisted and influenced each other in the experience narratives of our respondents. We embrace the idea of social distance as a material reality but seek to also reflect on the ways in which distance becomes "social" in relation to pandemic threat. First we consider the media engagements of our participants and the theme of "pandemic at a distance" that emerged in their persuasion narratives and the related prospect of narrative distanciation or alienation. We then reflect on the ways in which people spoke of distance as affording protection, or cordon sanitaire, but also how they made mention of the myths that supported this view of social distance and contagion. The last section of this chapter explores how people negotiated for forms of social distancing in domestic and working life and how they also admitted how these measures were difficult to implement, were partial, and were most probably ineffective. This chapter, therefore, supplies important insight into the cultural and social meanings of the narrative organization of social distance, a key intervention of the public health system in 2009 and currently in plans for future pandemics.

Pandemic at a Distance

The social meanings of distance and contagion are linked with a well-known trope that pandemic threat arises from somewhere else. Susan Sontag (1988) pointed out that cultural engagements with infectious diseases like syphilis were organized around notions of the foreign other as the source of contagion. Paula Treichler (1999), too, has discussed the categorization of those at risk of HIV—gay men, injecting drug users, sex workers—as a cultural method of assuring some distance from the threat implied by the virus. As we noted in the previous chapter, these cultural associations of other diseases layered how some of our participants engaged with the threat of pandemic influenza. Emily Martin's (1994) investigation of immunity in the United States took up questions of corporeal and social bodies defended against attack, among other versions of the science and culture of immunity. Mary Douglas's purity cosmology and framing of "matter out of place" (1966) addressed the cultural construction of boundaries and the related deepening of inside and outside identities and transgressive border crossings. One of the objectives of pandemic communications in 2009 was to persuade publics and individuals to think of themselves as at risk, if necessary, and therefore by implication to incorporate themselves into the cultural organization of contagion rationality and its connotations for social distance.

Wald has pointed out that contagion imaginaries depend on the inscription of the alien other in narrative. Influenza pandemics are iconic in this sense, since they are regularly named in the English-language media in ways that mark them as other and encroaching. Examples included "Asian flu" (1957–1958) and "Hong Kong flu" (1968–1969) (Kilbourne 2006). Influenza pandemics, partly because of their biological characteristics, have also been named according to species: "swine flu" (1976 and 2009) and "bird flu" (2004). The famous "Spanish flu" (1918–1919) followed this pattern though, as we have discussed, it has been argued that the name was coined because the Spanish news media documented the pandemic while English-language media self-censored in the interest of national unity in the time of war (Honigsbaum 2013). The northern-centric, emerging infectious disease narrative implicitly mobilizes the idea of the contagion from elsewhere, since the idea of a threat that is "emerging" implies that it comes from somewhere else.

As discussed, news media played a role in sustaining this idea of contagion coming into the lives of those at risk. The news media in the United Kingdom and Australia, from late April in 2009, circulated the story of the World Health Organization's announcement of a "public health emergency of international concern" and referred to the infections and fatalities in Mexico. This story of a contagious microbe emerging from elsewhere informed the narratives of those in our research who identified themselves as at risk. Sarah, who was discussed in chapter 2, depicted the scale-up of news media and the staging of the approaching threat:

> So initially, yes, I think it was just on the telly and it was, it just seemed to be every day it just seemed to be going up a level and up a level. And, you know,

for me I suppose the fear was just building and building with it, thinking, "Oh God, what's going to happen?" You know, "Is everybody going to, is it going to be real?" (Glasgow, 30s, Pregnant in 2009)

Sarah captured through her question, "What's going happen?," the sense that during the early stages of the pandemic, no one, experts included, could foresee how events would actually unfold. This portentous quality of pandemic storytelling lends it force and presumably explains why it is so often repeated across popular culture and the news media. As we have noted, a pandemic is an ideal story in the sense that it invites suspense and vigilance for what might happen next. Crucially, the spatialized implications of contagion are important. Sarah suggested, at first, distance from the pandemic. Her other question, "Is it going to be real?," indicated that, at least initially, Sarah regarded the pandemic as distant from her, geographically, but also in terms of her own health and risk. Her narrative on becoming persuaded into at-risk status, staged as a gradual realization, also mapped a pandemic traveling across distance into her life: coming to the United Kingdom, affecting particular groups and notably pregnant women, and then Sarah herself. Sarah's question and others like it from the narratives discussed previously suggested that accepting, eventually, risk status—taking on of the role of a character in the pandemic story—was a way of erasing the symbolic distance between mediatized, alien pandemic and personal experience. Claire also referred to this emerging pandemic idea:

I can remember seeing something about China and they were walking about with masks and it was on telly and I just thought, "What the hell is going on here?" and then they said that it had hit Britain. (Glasgow, 30s, Pregnant in 2009)

Claire associated China with these early reports, as did Sarah, though the pandemic was first notified in Mexico and soon after in the United States. It may be that China is metonymically linked with pandemic threat, echoing perhaps the more general Cold War resonance of pandemics (Martin 1994). Alternatively, news media on Avian influenza and SARS have involved countries in South East Asia, so references to China may have elided those stories with the news of the 2009 pandemic. Mary, who was introduced in the previous chapter, mentioned China and SARS, but was uncertain about the salience of each for the influenza pandemic, by her own admission. She spoke of the pandemic as, first, a distant reality:

INTERVIEWER: When you say that what are you thinking about, the swine flu or . . . ?

MARY: Well kind of both, I was thinking more of SARS actually when you saw it on telly with all the people and I don't want to say China because maybe it wasn't China but out . . . Asian kind of areas where everybody was wearing masks and going about and you thought, "I wonder if that'll come here and we'll have to do that?," because you just couldn't really visualize it. (Glasgow, 30s, Pregnant in 2009)

Mary reinforced the importance of communications and media for her pandemic experience when she said she "saw it on telly." But, like Sarah, Claire, and others in our research, news media articulations of the pandemic story reinforced the idea of contagion coming from elsewhere. Mary's thought to herself, "I wonder if it will come here?," indicated that our research participants had received and understood the "emerging from elsewhere" narrative on the pandemic.

There was also a sense in which the "from a distance" quality of news on the pandemic installed social distance between public health and its publics. Public health systems are highly reliant on communications and media to address their publics, particularly in situations when events unfold rapidly and unpredictably. Publics, too, are diverse and mobile. News media items from 2009 did often feature major political figures and chief public servants from health systems in ways that could be considered to have simulated interpersonal address, but these modes of communication are, strictly, not dialogical and therefore somewhat distancing. Those living highly medicalized lives with preexisting conditions and pregnant women gave the impression that they had access to the health system in ways that the healthy majority did not. It can be argued, therefore, that many, if not most, experienced the pandemic through communications and media and therefore their engagements with the public health system were also largely mediated and at a distance. Further, the telling and retelling of the pandemic story framed how publics engaged with public health experts who took the role of expert/hero in the dramatis personae of the pandemic narrative. As we have seen, too, this mediated, narrativized and distanced public health address to its publics was part of the "distant and emerging" theme of the personal experience narratives of people in our research. Efforts to explain and shape the risk reduction practice of social distancing, therefore, are complicated by the distancing effects of communications and media on pandemics and in particular the distancing quality of the nondialogical address of the public health system to its publics.

Sarah's, Claire's, and Mary's reflections and others like them on "pandemic at a distance" also have implications for conceptualizing narrative on pandemics and "narrative distanciation" (Czarniawska 2004). Narratives are often thought of as a means for forging identities, the establishment of social presence and the meaningful shaping of self and other relations (Andrews, Tamboukou, and Squire 2013). Narrative is often discussed in ways that assume that the narrator and their interlocutor are brought together in a quest for meaning as in some versions of narrative medicine (Greenhalgh 2006). But narrative need not always sustain connection. It can also alienate the narrator and the reader from each other, as we noted in the introduction to this chapter. It can be fashioned to create distance between narrator and audience and produce a kind of bidirectional othering and therefore work to produce "social" distance. Sarah's and Mary's reference to pandemic news on the "telly" and the note made by Claire and Mary of "China" as the place where the virus was emerging suggest how the H1N1 pandemic was at first a story of the distant other and only gradually one in which these interviewees came to see themselves. Mary posed the question, "I wonder if that'll come here and we'll have to do that?," which tells of physical distance but also of social separation. This distanciating quality of news stories is an important insight for the heralded turn to narrative persuasion in public health communications. Not all narratives are immediately persuasive, nor do they uniformly interpellate their subjects.

Cordon Sanitaire and Mythical Distance

The concept of a pandemic emerging from a distance was combined in interviews and focus groups with the age-old idea of enclosed, delimited space as a method of avoiding contagion. For example, respondents who lived on city fringes regarded their place of residence as itself a form of protection. For example, Deb, whom we introduced in the previous chapter, lived with her family on the urban fringe of Melbourne, and at the outbreak of the pandemic she had a newborn baby. When asked if she had taken any specific precautions at the time she responded:

> I don't think so. I don't think I thought it was a serious enough threat for our immediate vicinity. Yeah. I think that was the case 'cause I hardly ever

go to the city. More so I stay in my local area so I didn't think it was a threat. (Melbourne, 30s, New baby in 2009)

In this account, Deb signaled ideas of distance as protection and in particular the city as a source of the virus. Deb seemed to rely not on any change in her behavior but simply on the notional distance between herself and the pandemic, that is, a cordon sanitaire of physical and interpersonal separation.

Other people in our research spoke of going to greater lengths to establish social distance. Jenny and Simon were aged in their 50s and 60s and, like Deb, lived on a property in the urban fringe of Melbourne. Jenny, while generally healthy, was prone to chest infections, and Simon's health was somewhat compromised due to a chronic illness. As soon as they heard of the threat of the pandemic Jenny took immediate action to isolate her family:

SIMON: And when the previous sort of scare for the terrible influenza [in 2009] we certainly did modify our behavior. So we spent less time going out and far more of it was up to me to be sent out. Provisioning the house. So we filled up the pantry.
INTERVIEWER: So you filled up the pantry and avoided going out?
SIMON: To some degree. But I mean we sort of bought things so you buy flour so that you can make bread and all, that sort of thing, so if it really came to the crunch we could isolate ourselves. Yeah.
JENNY: But I don't think that anyone else that we know did. So we are just over, over cautious. (Melbourne, Jenny: 60s, Lung disease, Simon: 50s, Chronic illness)

Jenny and Simon gave the impression that when they heard of the pandemic they were poised in readiness and had made preparations to implement "isolation" if need be. Later when asked what she remembered the government doing Jenny said:

Well they told you not to panic. No need to overreact. They were worried about runs on the supermarkets and things like that. It was too late: we'd already done that. I certainly wouldn't take any notice of them saying not to do that. If I felt there was any chance of anything like that, I would do a run on the supermarket. But eventually they'd run out and you'd be up the creek.

SIMON: The World Health Organization put out sort of levels and they, their level was that you should stockpile food. So we did.

Jenny and Simon spoke of the media hype critique, which was a recurrent theme across interviews and focus groups, and Jenny's statement, "I certainly wouldn't take any notice," suggested mistrust, a theme we take up in chapter 8. Their preparations for self-isolation, not to protect others from infection but to close themselves off from contagion, has the air of the discourse of "doomsday preppers" (Paffenroth 2011, Zealand 2011). Their talk of social distancing suggests individualism, an effect of pandemic preparedness that we will revisit in the following chapter about immunity.

Others in our interviews and focus groups who lived in cities did not have the inbuilt social distance of people like Deb, Jenny, and Simon. Seeking out social distance under these circumstances was discussed, however. For example, Gill, discussed in chapter 3, became aware that the H1N1 infection had been notified among children at a local school:

GILL: Well given that there was flu at [school] and my son was three and he was at [childcare center], I pulled him out. So when my husband picked him up that day I was at work, I said, "Take him home. Give him a bath. Wash his clothes." I stopped sending him and I was one week off my maternity leave so I stopped work a week early. I didn't go to the supermarket. Didn't really mix.
INTERVIEWER: So really reduced your contact with people?
GILL: Very much so, yes.
INTERVIEWER: How did you manage to cope with that in terms of I s'pose the practicalities of life?
GILL: Well, I got groceries delivered online. We went out but to places like the Botanic Gardens and just tried to avoid shopping centers and movie theaters, and play groups. And, we did see family, but I did ask them to wash their hands when they came in. (Melbourne, 30s, Pregnant in 2009)

Gill's account of her response drew on the idea of social distance as enclosure of space and of the construction of protective distancing, even in the situation of the pandemic having emerged in the same neighborhood. Like other expectant mothers in our research, Gill gave an account that depicted her as a responsible parent: quick to act and decisive. Social distance for her appeared to have been adopted with some success for a limited time, despite the costs it might have incurred.

Gordon, who lived in outer Melbourne with lung disease, commented that Australia's geography and, in some respects, history, afforded protection:

GORDON: I think we're very lucky here. We are very isolated. There's not many of us.
INTERVIEWER: So you mean isolated as in Australia or as in this area?
GORDON: Well both. Australia and even our cities are isolated. I mean in Europe they're all on top of each other. So, Asia they're on top of each other. We're very lucky. Not so lucky anymore though because the world's getting closer and closer to us. There's millions of people coming and going from all over the world. And so we can't avoid it forever I don't think. I think we'll get it.
INTERVIEWER: So you think that distance helps Australians?
GORDON: Yeah, yeah. And I think we're pretty hardy stock too. I think it's a pretty harsh country and it's made our descendants pretty hard people, and good, strong, solid stock, basically, even though a lot of us are immigrants. I think it's the sort of country that, with that huge desert in the middle of it everything's gotta come through that almost to get to us. I think that helps. (Melbourne, 60s, Lung disease)

Gordon's account rather complexly referred to viruses and people coming from outside Australia, which, due to its separation from the world, was partly protected. He admitted, however, that the impossibility of his idea of enclosed space meant that the protective distance Australia had enjoyed was collapsing. His account therefore made reference to the other meaning of space that is implicit in the idea of a pandemic threat, that is, space as networked and traversable. He reasoned that in the face of the encroaching networked space of threat, resilient bodies, forged in the harsh Australian environment, could resist the pandemic. Informing this account, too, was the idea of Australia as "the lucky country," the title of a well-known book by Donald Horne (Horne 1964), which has become idiomatic in Australia, though, more recently, in an ironic sense. Gordon's account was therefore partly an expression of the material realities of geographic distance and partly a myth of Australia identity. Gordon's account, engaging with distance, pandemics, and identity as it did, staged also a narrative of Australia becoming a part of networked, global space. As we noted in chapter 1, Melbourne for a short period of time was a significant epicenter of H1N1 transmission, a feature of the pandemic's history that underlines the mythical quality to Gordon's reference to protective distance, but also indicates the preeminence of globally networked space for pandemic realities.

Gordon's narrative also drew on an implied and possibly racist othering of both Europeans and Asians, which referred to long-standing cultural anxiety regarding Australia's place in the world and the waves of migration that have made it what it is (Harris 2013). Both Sontag (1988) and Wald (2008), among others, have made the point that pandemic imaginaries help to construct relationships between self and threat from somewhere else—a social distanciation that can be stabilized in the figure of the other—often in ways that follow systems of caste, class, race, and in the case of H1N1, species, since the 2009 pandemic was typed as "swine" flu. This effect of pandemic storytelling is one reason why both Sontag and Wald ask for ethical responses to the social and cultural organization of pandemic narratives, as a matter of social redress and to overcome habits of thought that demonize the other.

Gordon's depiction of the resilient bodies and mentalities of Australians demonstrated that pandemic stories can be shaped around local myths of identity defined against the contagious other. But contradiction was also apparent. Gordon went on to argue that he lived apart from others, but also pointed out that his reliance on the myth of safe distance was exposed to him because of how he interacted with others in his daily life:

> You know where I live. This is the big smoke [referring to the small local township location of the interview]. Where I live is in the forest itself. And we're surrounded by forest. And we try to be self-sufficient. I would never stick my head out here [township location of the interview] again. But then I probably have to 'cause I love coming to have a cup of coffee and things like that, and going out. So I think it helps if you're isolated. When I was working, I'm still working there but when I am at [a local tourist attraction] I'm not isolated because, you know with all the tourists and what have you.

Gordon endorsed social distance as a method of protection, but he also acknowledged contradiction because he enjoyed social events that took him into places where he would be in contact with people and because his employment brought him into contact with travelers. While he may have built a cordon sanitaire between himself and the apparent source of contagion, elaborated with myths of Australian identity, his method was flawed and self-consciously so. It provided him with a sense of safety, diffusing pandemic threat and its fear-producing connotations, but at the same time was understood to be ineffective in an absolute sense. In this view, the reliance on the figure of the contagious other as a method of stabilizing social and physical distance, is itself unstable, prone to dissolution in the face of the admission of global networks and social interaction which makes life viable.

Negotiable and Partial Social Distance

Social distance was therefore instantiated in the spreading and encroaching threat narrative circulated in media and that informed the interpellation of the "at risk." Some of our respondents drew on social distance as a literalized and mythologized form of self-protection, though Gordon recognized perhaps in a self-effacing way, the illusions to which his method of cordon sanitaire was subject. People we spoke with also used social distance inventively, to develop localized arrangements at home, work, and in social life. These enactments of social distance were, however, partial and provisional and relied on cooperation with others. These stories attest to the complexities and challenges of taking precautions in the circumstances of everyday life.

Maude, who lived in Glasgow and was pregnant at the time of the pandemic in 2009, explained her engagement with the early communications and media in terms of pandemic distanciation we have discussed in connection with Sarah, Claire, and Mary. She went on to offer an account of a friend who had to self-isolate due to infection:

INTERVIEWER: We're going to go into public communications that you remembered . . . Can you go back in time to when it started?
MAUDE: I suppose from the news would've been the first that we heard about the couple that came back from Mexico or something? South America? And obviously they were, I think they were fairly local, they were Glasgow weren't they the couple that came back? I suppose it started from then. I then had a friend who then did have suspected swine flu. She was one of the earliest cases, and I know she was given Tamiflu and her whole family was given Tamiflu. But it was then at the stage when they'd stopped testing so she will now never know if that was actually swine flu that she had or whether it was just a very severe flu. But because of the time that it was, sort of early summer 2009 or one of the earliest cases it was just, well they were still giving Tamiflu to everybody and your whole family if you had it but they'd just stopped testing if they thought you had it. So I suppose that

was a bit like, "Oh this is actually getting a bit close to home, we now know somebody directly who you know is getting this."

INTERVIEWER: And at that point that stuck out as I suppose one of your first memories, what do you remember?

MAUDE: I suppose just that this is actually something that is going to affect us all. This isn't something that's going to be contained. This is going worldwide. This is everybody and I suppose then that we started looking at, "Right these are the symptoms." I do remember that time we all had coughs that seemed to last for, well months, two or three months, but that was the worst that we got. (Glasgow, 30s, Pregnant in 2009)

Maude's reference to "a bit close to home" underlined the idea of emerging threat and therefore the related idea of contagion flowing across distance. Like other pregnant women in our research Maude appeared to have been called into action. Her account also featured a story of assisting her quarantined friend in a manner that suggested the feminization of healthcare associated with pandemic influenza:

And I remember leaving pots of food under there [points outside]. We've got a trampoline in the back garden and I do remember making like big pans of soup and big pans of bolognaise sauce and stuff like that and going no further than just into their back door gate and leaving food parcels for them under their trampoline and saying like, "There you go!," because obviously the rest of the family needed to eat as well and obviously they were all taking Tamiflu, but they weren't ill. And just saying, "Right that's what we can do, but we're not actually coming in your house!" (laughs)

INTERVIEWER: And how did that feel?

MAUDE: It was strange not to be able to go in and help I suppose my initial reaction would've been, "Well I'll come in and help look after you or I'll come in and I'll cook in your house." Whereas you were just having to take that extra step and say well that's maybe, with having young children in our house, that's a risk too much. But I can cook and you obviously want to be able to help your friends out when you can.

INTERVIEWER: And how did you communicate with them?

MAUDE: Just through text messages and phone and I suppose that's it. That's the advantage of mobile phones and technology that we have.

Maude depicted herself as good neighbor and perhaps an ideal citizen of the pandemic response since she recognized the need to support the social isolation of her friend and family, but also that assisting them was a valuable form of care. This story is striking too for the importance of collaboration and signals that social distancing procedures call on social networks, neighbors and collectives, not only individuals.

Like Maude, Angela spoke of instituting some precautions in 2009. Angela lived in inner Melbourne, was also pregnant in 2009, and had a pragmatic response to the pandemic and her potentially heightened risk:

> I definitely tried to avoid people like that [anyone coughing or sneezing]. I think at one stage they were saying that people who'd been overseas so I kind of you know, did the mental calculation about who was likely to have been overseas and that sort of thing. And for a while just bunkered down. I think it was winter, wasn't it? Like autumn, coming into winter. So we didn't do a lot of socializing anyway, we kind of just cocooned up. Like not seeing anyone because it was cold and we'd kind of just hang out. And hung out with friends. We didn't do, basically we didn't do parties, but we obviously socialized with friends who came over and brought their kids, and had dinners and that sort of thing. More like one-on-one or family rather than going to a place with thirty families. We didn't do that. (Melbourne, 30s, Pregnant in 2009)

Angela provided a story of someone who had internalized the advice from public health experts and had accordingly attempted to moderate her risk of transmission through social distancing. There was a sense, though, that her approach was imperfect by her own admission, since she did report socializing with friends and family. She also provided a story of how she had negotiated to stay home from work during her pregnancy:

INTERVIEWER: So is that where you got most of your information?
ANGELA: Yes, yes. Most of it was from *The Age* [Melbourne broadsheet newspaper]. And I remember quite a few pieces that were very alarmist. But they were useful 'cause I actually took them in to show my boss and said, "Look," you know, "basically women are being told to work from home." And I did work from home a couple of times when no one was able to give me a lift. I thought they were quite useful.

INTERVIEWER: Very handy!

ANGELA: I know that other women at work also who were pregnant also relied on some of those quite alarmist articles to say, "Look, I'm not going in. I'm working from home." It gave everyone a bit of a break.

INTERVIEWER: And was the workplace supportive of that?

ANGELA: Yes, yes, you know. I worked in a big firm so, you know, they had procedures in place and they were all very worried about risk. But, you know, they had the odd person who was like, you know, "You women are just taking us for a ride." You know. They were very sexist and very conservative but they did worry about the level of risk.

Angela offered a story on the workplace and gender, providing insight into how the pandemic message made it possible for her and women like her to negotiate safer working practices for themselves during the pandemic. Her account indicated that news media hype could be turned to productive uses. Her story also underlined the interpersonal nature of the negotiation for social distancing since permission to stay home from work had to be sought and, it seemed, was established with some effort to persuade her employer into her way of thinking.

While Angela reported that she had been successful, many others, like Brigitte, introduced at the beginning of this chapter, were reluctant to avoid work and face the risks of negative judgement by employers. For example, Xavier who was in his 30s and lived in Sydney, noted: "I sort of feel obliged to go in [to work]. Yeah. So I always go in . . . unless I'm taking a holiday. I never take a sick day for anything' (Sydney, 30s, No disclosed health problems). These concerns over workplace reputation may have reflected desires to sustain good relationships with employers and therefore ensure continued employment and other benefits. It also appeared to be the case that asking for time off to manage illness attracted some resistance. Nicole, in her 20s and a healthcare worker who lived in inner Sydney with lung disease, related a story of one occasion when she attempted to negotiate time away from the workplace:

We have an aid on which is like the nurse who's on overnight. And she said to me, "Are you sure it's that bad?" And I said, "Yes, I'm quite sure." And she said, "Well it's not very good to call me at two o'clock in the morning and say you're sick." And I said, "Well you've got plenty of time to call an agency. You've got five hours." And she said, "Well, it's just a cough. It can't be that bad." And I said, "Oh yes you're a nurse, yes?" And she said, "Yes."

And I said, "Good. I'm a nurse too and I'm telling you it's that bad." And yeah . . . I'm not gonna argue with these people, "Would you like me to cough in your ear?" (Sydney, 20s, Lung disease)

Using reported dialogue to emphasize the dramatic tension of this event, Nicole revealed how her judgment was resisted and challenged. As we have indicated, too, it was apparent that attempts to perform social distancing were partial and incomplete. Cindy, who had lung disease, also made reference to social distancing with workmates and friends, but noted that her boyfriend was exempted:

I mean with like my peers and my colleagues we'll change our behavior but when I've got a partner, we don't change any of our behavior. We just figure well we're gonna catch it anyway so we won't change . . . like we don't separate for the week or, you know, live separately or what have you. So that's probably the only person in my life that we don't change behaviors for, who are sick. (Sydney, 20s, Lung disease)

Cindy was focused on protecting her health, but her account revealed her social distance strategy to have been flawed since protective distance from the source of an infection depended not only on her own practices but also on those of her partner. Cindy appeared to accept that her use of social distancing was limited, perhaps because, like many of our respondents she recognized that social distancing was of limited use in any case. Her account also underlined the framing of pandemic space as inescapably networked, if not through herself, then through her partner.

The improbable nature of social distancing was discussed in our interviews and focus groups. Diane, who lived in inner Melbourne and had a compromised immune system due to a recent illness, related a story of how her hospital had made efforts to protect others when she was found to have a possible infection with the H1N1 virus:

I had it [influenza] in the midst of chemotherapy treatment. And I was put into isolation, which is actually a good thing, because they didn't want other people to [be infected], 'cause you were in a ward full of people. And I felt really, really sick. But I felt pretty sick anyway so I wasn't particularly distinguishing until afterward that I actually felt so lousy because of the flu as well as the chemotherapy as well. (Melbourne, 50s, Severe illness in 2009)

Later in her interview, Diane was asked how influenza could be avoided. Her response indicated that the management of transmission in "real life" was not easy:

> I'm not quite sure how [to avoid influenza]. From what I know of how it's passed on, it's actually through like droplets in the air. So if somebody sneezed or coughed, or something? It's not as if people go around deliberately passing on the flu. I s'pose isolation is one way of avoiding it but it's very hard to achieve isolation in real life, isn't it? And I s'pose if you've been in really good health, you're less likely to catch it. I imagine you're more likely to be able to fight it off or get rid of it quickly. So I don't know. But I think vaccinations have actually reduced the flu. So that preventative stuff must work in some ways. So to that degree I think we can avoid catching it if you take those precautions. But it's not likely guaranteed. The strains keep changing and, also, your system might be up or down. You might be vulnerable, you know.

Diane's account indicated awareness of the range of nonpharmaceutical and pharmaceutical methods used to mitigate and treat infection, including social distance. She noted, perhaps reflecting on her experience in hospital, that social distance was effective, but also that, in daily life at least, it was hard to achieve. Through reference to the idea of "system might be up or down," Diane's account also made telling reference to the importance of one's immune system for the management of infection, since methods of social distancing were likely to be ineffective. This resort to immunity in the face of the failures of social distance and other methods of controlling the spread of the virus revealed a belief that the microbe would breach space and barriers and therefore enter the body. In this situation, the ability of the body to deal with the infection became important. Diane's reference to vaccines underlined this idea of bodily resilience in the face of the inevitable incursion of the virus. This point of view and others like it were indicative of networked pandemic space and a mobile virus. Distance and boundaries and related notions of enclosed space were seen as untenable. The importance of immunity in the open, networked spaces of pandemic threat is further elaborated in the next chapter.

The idea that social distancing methods were unlikely to be effective in the long run was a recurring theme in interviews and focus groups. In this quotation, Roslyn, a retiree in her 60s living with her husband on the outskirts of Melbourne, made reference to an experience where she thought she may have been exposed to seasonal influenza:

> I was just very careful about what we did and where we went. But it's a bit like many, many years ago they said that the communists were coming. Well we're still waiting. So I think for people to be aware of the severity of these things is important. But I think there's very little the general public can do apart from taking care of themselves and using any sort of technique that is a barrier. I mean I really don't know that there's anything you can do. To be aware, as I say, and don't travel overseas if you don't have to, or don't get in, you know, a confined space like a plane.... Last year I went on an excursion with a community group and the guy behind me had the most awful cough and cold. He was taking this pill and that pill. And he said, "Oh have you got any water? I need to take my antibiotics." I said, "Well you're not getting my water bottle! I'll get a cup but you're not having my bottle." Well two weeks later I had it. Being in a confined space is not good. (Melbourne, 60s, No disclosed health problems)

Roslyn likened government warnings on the pandemic to the unrealized moral panics of the past and, in particular, Cold War discourse (Martin 1994), and signaled the skepticism that characterized the responses of people in our research. Her reference to "antibiotics" showed that immunity was also a consideration in the management of infection, echoing Diane, already discussed. The story Roslyn provided of the inevitability of infection indicated belief that infection was difficult to avoid, even if one was careful about social interaction, casting doubt on the advice from public health. Her account also made reference to different kinds of spaces implied in pandemic threat. There was the notion of the "communists were coming" from somewhere else and the "confined" space of the bus. There was also the intimate space of touch implied in the sharing of the water. These different kinds of spaces where contagion was implicated were used to demonstrate the complexity of social life and the improbability of being able to avoid infection.

Sarah from Glasgow, who was introduced in chapter 2, spoke of the virtual impossibility of avoiding influenza short of shutting oneself away from society:

> To avoid catching it? . . . I don't think so, I really don't think so. I think you can try and do things to minimize your chances of getting it, but I don't

think you can avoid catching it altogether. I think you can do things like you know . . . the hand washing thing and just being a wee bit more aware of your like you know, I'm always trying to get [Sarah's son] to cover his mouth when he's coughing and sneezing and using a tissue and all that sort of stuff. So you can do all these things, but I don't think you can completely avoid getting it altogether. It's an airborne virus is it not? So you're going to breathe it, you know short of locking yourself up in a room . . . .

Sarah's example signaled how an impractical—even absurd—social isolation would be the only guarantee of preventing transmission. These various points of view of the limited and even improbable nature of the social distancing method foreshadow our next chapter, on immunity, which explores how people were compelled to reflect on how to fabricate bodily resilience to influenza because it was generally believed that the virus was not possible to avoid in the real world for any length of time, except under the "impossible" situation of total social isolation.

Pandemic preparedness and response documents refer to social distancing as one method for moderating the spread of the virus in the period of time in which scientists and technicians search for and produce a viable vaccine. Social distancing is not seen as a panacea, though it is also understood as a reserve power of public health authority that could be extended in more rigorous ways in the case of a severe public health emergency, as was done in Toronto for SARS in 2003. Publics understood social distancing in these ways and contended with its limitations. They were also aware of the other rationality of distance as a network and flow of people and microbes that interrupted and complicated efforts to create social distance in the mode of enclosure and protection from contagion.

The accounts we have discussed in this chapter do not suggest subjects who had complacently thrown off advice regarding social distancing. There were indications of engaged subjects, inventively negotiating and appropriating the social distancing message in ways that worked for them and their personal circumstances. What has been construed as a weak enactment of social distance in survey research (Mitchell et al. 2011) could also be seen as the expression of the practical problems related to social relations with others and the negotiation of the institutions of everyday life and, in particular, the workplace. These insights are important for shaping messages for the general public with regard to nonpharmaceutical methods of disease control. The mixture of physical and social spatializations of pandemic threat underlines in another way the entanglement of media, pandemic, and lived experience.

The analysis we have presented was sensitive to the contagion metaphor, which gives narrative on pandemic some of its potency. In this regard, advice to enact social distance coexists with other meanings of social distance, including media depictions of emerging microbial threat, myths of enclosed space erased by networked space, and the somewhat alienating quality of pandemic threat. Social distance, informed as it is by the metaphorical potential of contagion, is found to be deeply and complexly enmeshed with the cultural organization of responses to microbial threat.

This chapter has employed the contagion metaphor to explore personal experience narratives on the enactment of social distance. Contagion, bridging as it does politics and biomedicine, provides a useful lens on the biopolitical ramifications of public health efforts to shape the behaviors of individuals and populations. In keeping with this method of analysis and as has been foreshadowed in this and previous chapters, the next chapter turns to talk on immunity: another political-biomedical metaphor that is important to public health efforts and to pandemic narrative.

References

Andrews, M, M Tamboukou, and C Squire, eds. 2013. *Doing narrative research, second edition*. London: Sage.
Appadurai, A. 2013. *The future as cultural fact: Essays on the global condition*. London: Verso.
Australian Department of Health. 2014. *Australian health management plan for pandemic influenza*. Canberra: Commonwealth of Australia.
Australian Government Department of Health and Ageing. 2011. *Review of Australia's health sector response to pandemic (H1N1) 2009: Lessons identified*. Canberra: Commonwealth of Australia.
Baehr, P. 2005. "Social extremity, communities of fate, and the sociology of SARS." *Archives of European Sociology* 46 (2):179–211.
Butler, D. 2014. "Tamiflu report comes under fire: Conclusions of the stockpiling of antiviral drugs challenged." *Nature* 508 (April 24):439.
Cauchemeza, S, A Bhattaraib, T Marchbanks, R Faganb, S Ostroffc, N Ferguson, D Swerdlow, and the Pennsylvania H1N1 working group. 2011. "Role of social networks in shaping disease transmission during a community outbreak of 2009 H1N1 pandemic influenza." *Proceedings of the National Academy of Sciences* 108 (7):2825–2830.
Centers for Disease Control and Prevention. 2009. "Outbreak of swine-origin Influenza A (H1N1) virus infection—Mexico, March–April 2009." *Morbidity and Mortality*

Weekly Report 58 (April 30):1–3. Accessed December 18, 2015. http://www.cdc.gov/mmwr/preview/mmwrhtml/mm58d0430a2.htm.

Cohen, R, and P Kennedy. 2000. *Global sociology*. Houndmills Palgrave.

Collier, S, and A Lakoff. 2015. "Vital systems security: Reflexive biopolitics and the government of emergency." *Theory, Culture & Society* 32 (2):19–51.

Czarniawska, B. 2004. *Narratives in social science research*. London: Sage.

Douglas, M. 1966. *Purity and danger: An analysis of concepts of pollution and taboo*. London: Routledge.

Foucault, M. 2007. *Security, territory, population: Lectures at the College de France, 1977–1978*. New York: Picador.

Greenhalgh, T. 2006. *What seems to be the trouble? Stories in illness and healthcare*. Oxford: Radcliffe Publishing.

Harris, A. 2013. *Young people and everyday multiculturalism*. New York: Routledge.

Health Protection Scotland. 2010. *The pandemic of Influenza A(H1N1) infection in Scotland 2009–2010: A report on the health protection response*. Glasgow: Health Protection Scotland.

Hine, D. 2010. *The 2009 Influenza pandemic: An independent review of the UK response to the 2009 influenza pandemic*. London: Pandemic Flu Response Review Team, Cabinet Office.

Honigsbaum, M. 2013. "Regulating the 1918–19 pandemic: Flu, stoicism and the Northcliffe Press." *Medical History* 57 (2):165–185. doi: http://dx.doi.org/10.1017/mdh.2012.101.

Horne, D. 1964. *The lucky country*. Camberwell: Penguin.

Kilbourne, E. 2006. "Influenza pandemics of the 20th century." *Emerging Infectious Diseases* 12 (1):9–14.

Lakoff, Andrew. 2015. "Real-time biopolitics: The actuary and the sentinel in global public health." *Economy and Society* 44 (1):40–59. doi: 10.1080/03085147.2014.983833.

Martin, E. 1994. *Flexible bodies: Tracking immunity in American culture from the days of polio to the age of AIDS*. Boston: Beacon Press.

Mitchell, T, DL Dee, CR Phares, et al. 2011. "Non-pharmaceutical interventions during an outbreak of 2009 pandemic influenza A (H1N1) virus infection at a large public university, April–May 2009." *Clinical Infectious Diseases* 52 (Suppl 1):S138–S145.

Morse, S. 1995. "Factors in the emergence of infectious diseases." *Emerging Infectious Diseases* 1 (1):7–15.

Paffenroth, K. 2011. "Zombies as internal fear or threat." In *Generation zombie: Essays on the living dead in modern culture*, edited by S Boluk and W Lenz, 18–26. Jefferson, NC: McFarland.

Public Health England. 2014. *Pandemic influenza response plan, 2014*. London: Public Health England.

Rutter, PD, OT Mytton, BM Ellis, and L Donaldson. 2014. "Access to the NHS by telephone and Internet during an influenza pandemic: An observational study." *BMJ Open* 4:e004174. doi:10.1136/bmjopen-2013-004174.

Sanford, S, and S Ali. 2005. "The new public health hegemony: Response to severe acute respiratory syndrome (SARS) in Toronto." *Social Theory & Health* 3:105–125.

Scholte, J 2000. *Globalisation*. Houndmills Palgrave.

Singer, M. 2016. "The spread of Zika and the potential for global arbovirus syndemics." *Global Public Health* 12 (1):1–18. doi: 10.1080/17441692.2016.1225112.

Sontag, S. 1988. *AIDS and its metaphors*. London: Penguin.

Treichler, P. 1999. *How to have theory in an epidemic: Cultural chronicles of AIDS.* Durham: Duke University Press.

UK Review on Antimicrobial Resistance. 2016. *Tackling drug-resistant infections globally: Final report and recommendations.* London: Wellcome Trust and HM Government.

Wald, P. 2008. *Contagious: Cultures, carriers, and the outbreak narrative.* Durham: Duke University Press.

World Health Organization. 2003. "Update 49—SARS case fatality ratio, incubation period." Accessed December 18, 2015. http://www.who.int/csr/sarsarchive/2003_05_07a/en/.

World Health Organization. 2011. *Implementation of the International Health Regulations (2005): Report of the Review Committee on the Functioning of the International Health Regulations (2005) in relation to Pandemic (H1N1) 2009. Report by the Director-General.* Geneva: World Health Organization.

Zambon, M. 2014. "Developments in the treatment of severe influenza: Lessons from the pandemic of 2009 and new prospects for therapy." *Current Opinion in Infectious Diseases* 27 (6):560–565. doi: 10.1097/QCO.0000000000000113.

Zealand, C. 2011. "The national strategy for zombie containment: Myth meets activism in post 9/11 America." In *Generation zombie: Essays on the living dead in modern culture,* edited by S Boluk and W Lenz, 231–247. Jefferson, NC: McFarland.

5
Immunity

So you really can't avoid it. You can eat well, sleep well. You can do all those sorts of things to give your immune system a chance to throw it off. I mean basically there's really no barrier that will ever stop you getting a cold or the flu, or whatever. (Roslyn, Melbourne, 60s, No disclosed health problems)

Talk of immunity was a prominent theme of the interviews and focus groups we conducted. The ease with which the virus passed between people and the rapidity of its spread over vast distances appeared to lead our research participants to say, as Roslyn did in the above quotation, that infection with the virus was not practically avoidable. In connection with the apparent inevitability of infection, respondents dwelt on the capacity of their bodies to cope with the virus. Immunity was only ever implied in public health communications and news media on the 2009 pandemic, despite its relevance for social distancing, hygiene, antivirals and vaccines. The planning documents that guided the public health response to the pandemic made scant reference to immunity in general and personal immune systems as methods of dealing with a global pandemic, though strictly speaking, vaccination is indeed a biotechnological manipulation of the human immune response. Given that it was implicated in the management of pandemic influenza, the lack of direct reference to immunity gave it a taken-for-granted status in planning documents, communications, news media, and the accounts of our respondents. Immunity per se was not originally on our agenda in interviews and focus groups, though it soon became obvious to us that it was important.

Immunity, like contagion, is a richly nuanced metaphor that gives pandemic narratives some of their potency. As Wald noted, notions of immunity are implied in stories, films, and television programs on viral catastrophe and alien invasion (2008). H.G. Wells's *War of the Worlds*, serialized in magazines in 1897, was an early example of the narrative potential of immunity. This well-known and much revisited story featured an alien invasion that was eventually brought down by the Earth's microbial life. Wells's book was written in the decades after Koch's observations of microbes, new explanations of disease pathogenesis, and the birth of the biomedical science of infectious diseases and related public health interest in contagion and hygiene (Pelling 1997). The title of Wells's book referred to the battle between the alien invaders and humanity, but it also referred to the ceaseless struggle of life on Earth involving microbes. As the final pages of the story have it, humanity had learned to live with microbes across millennia, unlike the newly arrived Martians, implying that biological survival is a lengthy and hard-won negotiation of coexistence. As we explain in what follows, narrative on immunity emerged in the accounts of people in our research when they reflected on the pandemic influenza virus, which they understood to escape efforts to control its incursion into society and individual bodies, forcing a focus on surviving, as opposed to preventing, infection.

Immunity is also a common and widely advertised consumer object, featuring in, for example, probiotic yogurts, superfoods, vitamins, and even mindfulness courses and self-help books on happiness and well-being (Burges Watson, Moreira, and Murtagh 2009, Koteyko 2009, Nerlich and Koteyko 2008). Honigsbaum (2013), in his discussion of media on the 1918–1919 influenza pandemic, noted how advertising of the period also articulated ideas of immunity. For example, the drink Bovril was advertised as a product that could "prevent influenza and colds by fortifying the system against their attacks" (2013, page 176), indicating that immunity was offered as a technology to repel the other, echoing as Honigsbaum argued, the war footing of Britain and allied nations. Contemporary advertising for Yakult makes reference to the idea of friendly bacteria, raising the prospect of microbial life as both useful and harmful to human life (Koteyko 2009). An Australian YouTube advertisement for surface cleaners was titled "*Dettol Mission for Health: The Strength of a Single Mum—See Nicole's Story*" and embedded the use of surface cleaners in a triumphal narrative on motherhood under conditions of adversity (Dettol 2013). The video featured a storyline where Nicole's children played "stuck in the mud," caught bugs in the garden, and read a children's illustrated book on bugs. The video ends with some frames of the family cleaning the house where the surface cleaner figures seamlessly as the natural adjunct to hygienic and harmonious domestic life protected from the "bug-life" that surrounds it.

Advertising like this depends on a tacit knowledge of immunity and related notions of contagion, combining therefore two of the powerful metaphors of narrative on microbial threat. *Nicole's Story* also suggests the feminization of labor on microbial threat, echoing comments in chapter 4 and prefiguring chapter 6, when we explore in more detail pandemic influenza and the gendering of healthcare.

The biopolitical, narrative, and consumer resonances of immunity are suggestive of "immunity culture." Our respondents provided many accounts of how they had experienced the pandemic through communications and news media, sometimes figuring their accounts as a gradual persuasion into the position of someone who might be at risk of the pandemic, particularly the pregnant women in our research. Gerlach and Hamilton (2014) have written of what they refer to as "pandemic culture," drawing together the variety of media forms that support narratives and narrative practices on the idea of a pandemic. Notable efforts include the CDC's use of zombie narratives and images to amplify the effectiveness of interventions on pandemic preparedness in the general public (Nasiruddin et al. 2013), and related efforts to combine expert knowledge with popular culture to fashion the edutainment genre of science and health communications. As we argue in what follows, immunity is so taken-for-granted yet axiomatic that it seems likely that pandemic culture is one, albeit important, intensification of the more general immunopolitics in affluent countries of the Global North.

In what follows, we explore the immunity talk of our respondents as it emerged in response to questions of how and whether or not pandemic influenza can be avoided. Our analysis reprises talk on social distancing in light of immunity, where respondents and in particular those with lung disease spoke of the impracticality and undesirability of social distancing and in that context spoke of immunity as the primary biomedical technology of their response to pandemic influenza. We discuss, also, the manner in which respondents spoke of acting on and acquiring their immunity as a matter of building corporeal vitality through consumer products and through productive communion with microbes. This chapter also considers the ways in which choice articulated through immunity deepened individualism in the public response to pandemic influenza and therefore accentuated problems for efforts to mobilize altruistic practices, such as herd immunity, in pandemic preparedness and response.

The Resort to Immunity

Talk on immunity emerged in our interviews and focus groups when we asked respondents to reflect on how they thought they could avoid pandemic influenza. Our questions were designed to draw out public perspectives on the recommended pandemic influenza mitigation strategies such as social distancing and hygiene and relatedly to explore perspectives on antivirals and vaccines as methods of pandemic influenza control. It became clear to us, however, that in response to questions on pandemic influenza control, respondents acknowledged that avoidance was not practical and, therefore, focused on how well their body might cope with infection, if need be.

As we have discussed in a previous publication (Davis et al. 2016), this narration of bodily resilience to infection accommodated the scientific complexities of immunity, including the biomedical definition of immunity as a system of cellular recognition of self and not self, and network immunity, that is, the idea that immunity depends on the productive relations of self and not self. These ways of speaking of immunity were combined with the idea of immunity as a personal acquisition open to reflexive management, or "choice" immunity, as we have called it. Donna Haraway has pointed out that immunity is a scheme for the biopolitical organization of self and other (1999, page 204). Emily Martin (1994) argued that the science of immunity and political economy in the United States have constituted each other. Drawing on these biopolitical readings, Ed Cohen (2009) has argued that the Latin root, *munis*, is revealing of the social and political underpinnings of "immunity." "Munis" is an ancient term that referred to a form of financial obligation to others with political and juridical connotations. Immunity, therefore, marked the circumstances where one's duty to others was suspended. As Cohen has shown, this political meaning of immunity was bound up with the emergence of an autonomous subject in the emerging political discourse of the early modern period. Biomedical immunity draws on this concept of self-definition to explain how some cells in the body have the capacity to identify and destroy foreign cells. Cohen's argument, however, and that of Haraway and Martin, is that the political symbolism of immunity is drawn into biomedical immunity to give it an intensely biopolitical resonance. As with the biomedical uses of the contagion metaphor to help explain germ theory noted in the previous chapter, immunity is a political concept that helps to construct biomedical knowledge, though in the mode of New Materialism, it can also be said that biological immunity has helped to constitute how political immunity is understood (Jamieson 2015). Immunity, however, implicates the body more directly than does contagion, since it dwells on the infection within—the "milieu interieur" as Cohen calls it (2009, page 239)—and as we will see in the discussion to follow, on manipulable, corporeal resilience and vitality.

Immunity, biomedical and otherwise, is also more complex than the simple idea of self defined against the other. Biological research shows that immunity is, as yet, a not fully understood interactive system of the body, microbes, and the bodies of others. Auto-immune disorders—where the body attacks itself—and microchimerism—where fetal cells continue to live in the mother's body after birth—show that the self can be alien to the self in some circumstances and that self and other can live together productively, too (Martin 2010). As we discussed in chapter 4 in relation to social distance, narrative on enclosed space coexisted with narrative on networked space since interconnections with others were necessary to social existence. Foucault (2007) and others have argued that the security of the social is found, not through delimitation and separation, but in the productive flows of goods, people, ideas, and, as will become apparent in what follows, microbial life, too.

This extract from Lola's interview was exemplary of talk on immunity from our research. Lola, who was in her 60s and lived in Melbourne without any disclosed illness, reflected on how the media had alerted her to the pandemic, like many of our respondents, but also that influenza was not readily amenable to biomedical intervention. Immunity, therefore, was necessary:

INTERVIEWER: So how have you come to learn about influenzas and particularly these pandemics when they come about?
LOLA: I think, really, majorly media and I think with the difference between say a cold and a flu, and then when you get treatment for a flu the fact that you can't, if you go and it's a viral flu there's absolutely nothing the doctors can do about that. But once it becomes an infection, a secondary infection, then they can treat that if it is in your lungs or wherever. Well I've understood that really through my background a little bit in medical work.
INTERVIEWER: And can you remember what sorts of things you've heard in the media?

LOLA: It's hugely alarming. Hugely alarming. It was. I think there's enormous fear in the community about it. And when we saw on the TV in Asia wasn't it? You know, that was really quite frightening I thought.

INTERVIEWER: How did you react to those messages?

LOLA: Oh I was quite concerned. I was very concerned. Because I feel that I've got a reasonably good handle on things as far as health and what to do, and I just think experiential learning has taken place, right. So I feel fairly confident that I know avoidance and I jump onto it straight away. Because I think that's the best way. Build up your immune system. So my idea was always building your immune system so that you're strong and if you're infected then your system is already stronger to cope with it than if you're working 80 hours a week drinking yourself silly at the weekend and smoking heaps of packets of cigarettes. You're just in a better position. Right? So I just kind of work on that basis I guess. So worried, yes, which is where I would feel at that time, for instance, if someone had said to me," We'll go and watch an indoor basketball match. There's going to be 5,000 people there." I would have said, "No." I wouldn't have minded. I would just happily say, "Oh look, no, I don't think so." But I didn't go around sort of in a panicked state, but I just felt it's a sensible decision—this isn't going to last forever. (Melbourne, 60s, No disclosed health problems)

Lola's account replayed the idea that the media hyped the pandemic and that, for a time in 2009, there was some anxiety about what might happen. It also referenced the idea of the pandemic as emerging elsewhere. Her account presented the idea that ensuring one is as healthy as possible is a key way of dealing with infection in combination with what appeared to be an admission of the value of social distancing. Important in Lola's account was the segue from news media on the pandemic to immunity, which suggested that messages to take action with regard to the impending emergency mobilized publics to think of how to bolster their health to cope with infection. In their research on public perceptions of colds and influenzas, Prior et al. (2011) found that their research participants made copious reference to immunity, indicating that bodily resilience was seen as an important resource in the ongoing struggle with microbes. Lundgren (2015) found that personal immunity also figured in the written accounts of colds and influenza generated by older Swedish people.

Our respondents, however, did not see that it was possible in the long run to avoid pandemic influenza. In this example, Roslyn, introduced in chapter 4 and at the beginning of this chapter, commented that measures could be taken to avoid infection, but that these were not likely to work in the long run:

INTERVIEWER: Do you think it's possible to avoid catching the flu?
ROSLYN: Well probably not. Well that depends again on, on how you live, how many people you come in contact with. Between us we've got a lot of friends and they know that if they've got a cold or the flu, they do not visit us because they will not be welcome. And that's our way of avoiding it coming into the house. So people know that if they are going to come and visit us and they have got a cough or otherwise if they do come and they've got a cold, I'll say, "Sorry..." I mean that's a way of protecting ourselves here but there's no way, you can't sort of... well you could wander around with a mask but it's not going to stop somebody sneezing on you in the supermarket or in the tram, or whatever. So you really can't avoid it. You can sort of eat well, sleep well. You can do all those sorts of things to give your immune system a chance to throw it off. I mean basically there's really no barrier that will ever stop you getting a cold or the flu, or whatever. (Melbourne, 60s, No disclosed health problems)

Like Lola, Roslyn argued that infection was inevitable in social life. Social distancing and hygiene were seen to provide some form of protection but not in an absolute sense. Roslyn reasoned, too, that along with the public health–sanctioned methods of social distancing and hygiene, rest and diet and therefore a more resilient corporeal self were elements of an effective response to pandemic influenza. In an interview in Scotland, Maude, whom we introduced in the previous chapter, made a similar comment:

INTERVIEWER: Do you think you can avoid the flu?
MAUDE: No, I don't think so. I think you can take measures to help with your hygiene and disposing of tissues carefully, and I suppose that's what you can do, but I suppose when you send your kids out to nursery, if they're going to get it, they're going to get it. If you travel on a bus you don't know who you sit next to. If you go on holiday you don't know who you sit next to. I don't think you can take every element out of it. I think that, yeah, you can reduce your risks, but you can't eliminate them all. I suppose I'm very much, "If you're going to get it you're going to get it," and just try and keep fit and healthy generally so that if you do get these things then you're

better equipped to fight them off you know. And I think I'm sure I read this somewhere that children need to have six colds in their first year to develop their immune system and part of me thinks that some illness, we do need some illness, that's what keeps us fit and healthy most of the time. So we have to build up our immune systems and we have to have some exposure otherwise how do you know what to fight against? (Glasgow, 30s, Pregnant in 2009)

Maude's account repeated the pattern of Lola's and Roslyn's. In the face of a question regarding whether influenza could be prevented, they each turned to embodied resilience, expressed in talk on immunity and immune systems. Their accounts reiterated points we raised in the previous chapter in connection with the impractical qualities of social distancing methods. These were seen as methods that could reduce risk, but not entirely, given the necessities of social interaction.

Social surveys conducted at the time of the 2009 pandemic found generally moderate to poor levels of reported compliance with the social distancing and hygiene measures advocated by public health authorities (Mitchell et al. 2011, Rubin et al. 2009, Seale et al. 2009). Based on the accounts of Lola, Roslyn, and Maude and others in our research, it was apparent that the nonpharmaceutical methods of infection control are endorsed but not understood to be protective in a practical, ongoing sense. In the face of the low perceived efficacy of the nonpharmaceutical methods, our respondents were encouraged to speak of their immunity even though immunity, and by implication bodily resilience, was only obliquely implicated in the communications strategies of public health. Immunity is the already and always present, subaltern technology of pandemic influenza preparedness and control.

The importance of immunity to our respondents was consistent with the machinery of pandemic preparedness and control, which did not aim to prevent influenza in an absolute sense since it is well known that influenza infection spreads easily (CDC 2014). This significance of immunity suggested, too, a presiding narrative of pandemic influenza as not strictly amenable to human action apart from what could be done to position corporeal resilience in the most favorable way. This pattern existed across the Australian and Scottish interviews and focus groups and across our different groups of the vulnerable and healthy, suggesting that the resort to immunity is widespread in those countries.

"You Can't Live in a Bubble"

The immunity talk sustained by our interviewees was complicated by reference to the idea that it was not possible or desirable to "live in a bubble." Lola, Roslyn, Maude, and others recognized that infection was difficult to resist. The metaphor of "can't live in a bubble" was used by respondents in our research with lung disease to explain, like Lola, Roslyn, Maude, and others, how influenza infection was difficult to avoid, but with the added sense of the significant risk faced by those with respiratory illness. The "can't live in a bubble" metaphor marked, therefore, vulnerability, but also resistance to this positioning. It suggested the importance of social contacts and networks to everyday life and a commitment on the part of people with lung disease to sustain their social lives. "Can't live in a bubble" referred to social life, but as we will see was also taken to imply that biological, and specifically immunological, life was not possible separated from others.

In this example, Archie, an older interviewee from Sydney with lung disease, used the bubble idea to reflect on avoiding flu infection:

INTERVIEWER: Do you think it's possible to avoid catching the flu in any way?
ARCHIE: No, I don't think it's possible to avoid catching it. I mean to avoid catching it you would have to live in a bubble. And I mean they don't even really know how it's spread. That's only from what I've read.
INTERVIEWER: Just on the Internet? Or—
ARCHIE: Yeah, on the Internet. On the American side of it. I mean you can go into a room where a person coughs once, and you could walk out of there, and 24 hours later you've got it. So I don't think you'll ever stop people from catching it. (Sydney, 60s, Lung disease)

Archie expressed the view shared by Lola, Roslyn, and Maude, but he couched it in the terminology that drew attention to the specific way in which he, as someone with lung disease, chose to live with microbial threat. Alex, living with lung disease, echoed Archie: "You can't live in a bubble . . . You gotta get out there" (Sydney, 30s). He signaled that it was imperative for him to stay engaged with others. Mitzi, living in Sydney and with lung disease, used the bubble metaphor after the interviewer asked her how she had responded to the pandemic:

INTERVIEWER: Can you remember the swine flu epidemic in 2009? How did you feel at that time about your health?

MITZI: I wasn't too worried about it but I must say my family was quite worried.

INTERVIEWER: For you personally or just general?

MITZI: For me personally. They were sort of like, "Well, you know, don't go anywhere and don't . . . ." My mum's like, she'll take like those Dettol wipes, when you touch a shopping trolley like wipe the shopping trolley. And I said, "I don't wanna be too pedantic." It looks like a germ freak. But they're worried that something like that can so easily just get you down.

INTERVIEWER: Did you do anything differently for that? Did you like get an extra jab or stock-up on any sanitizer and Dettol wipes?

MITZI: I don't think so. We're pretty careful anyway. Like I think we're pretty on top of . . . I think we've got a good balance of not going overboard and we can't live in a bubble. . . . But also not being slap-happy. Not too relaxed. Like we wouldn't go somewhere in close, confined spaces with lots of kids coughing and that sort of stuff. When the kids go to birthday parties my husband tries to take them. Like to those parties with everyone running around with all their germs. But we try not to live in a bubble. (Sydney, 30s, Lung disease)

Mitzi's account expressed worry over self-presentation that resonated with the "Be alert, not alarmed" theme of expert advice on the pandemic in 2009. Public health systems the world over sought out the "Be alert, not alarmed" message, which Briggs and Nichter characterized as the "Goldilocks" message (2009). Mitzi's "Goldilocks" message of "not too complacent and not too anxious self-presentation" reflected the balance that "Be alert, not alarmed" aimed to establish between preparing citizens for an emergency without them becoming overly anxious. In her interview, too, Mitzi referred to the management of social distance as we discussed in chapter 4, but also the idea that performing social isolation in the extreme was detrimental to social life. Later in her interview, Mitzi made a link between the bubble metaphor and immunity when the interviewer asked her how the risk of infection could be reduced:

Just your hand washing and using tissues and throwing them out. There's so many people that wipe their nose and then go and touch something or if you go to Woolworth's and you look at the people that wipe their nose with their tissue, put the tissue back in their pocket and then touch the cash register and hand your money. Like just little things like that. If you actually watch people, we're kind of gross. You know? Most of the time it's fine. Like you can't live in a bubble and you can't live in a sterile environment or you won't have an immune system at all.

Notable in this quotation was how Mitzi expanded on the need for connection with others, not only in terms of social life, but also in the interest of her health. According to Mitzi, lack of social interaction and therefore sterility would harm her immune system. Immunity, then, was understood to be in productive exchange with social and therefore microbial life.

The appearance of the bubble metaphor in the accounts of people with lung disease was suggestive of collective identity; a shared set of meanings of how to live with lung disease. The bubble metaphor indicated a form of biological citizenship in the sense of identity formed around a specific diagnosis (Petryna 2003, Rose and Novas 2005). We recruited people with lung disease from community-support groups, so it seems likely that we tapped into proto-pandemic citizenship mapped onto existing support structures.

The bubble metaphor was also suggestive of popular culture narrative, since it referenced the 1976 TV film *The Boy in the Plastic Bubble* (Kleiser 1976). This film depicted the life of a child whose immune system was so fragile that no contact with others could be risked: hence life in a plastic bubble. One theme of this film was the loss of humanity associated with living this way. When our interviewees used the bubble metaphor they gestured toward the difficulties, even impossibilities, of life out of contact with others. They also, implicitly and explicitly, brought in ideas of immunity and their relationships with immunity culture and related practices of self.

Choice Immunity

Also implied in narrative on the value of immunity was its status as a feature of the body open to reflexive management and that its existence and utility depended on the agential subject of immunity culture. This framing of immunity was consistent with the consumer-oriented currents of immunity and cohered with contemporary forms of biomedicine that give emphasis to self-care and autonomous action (Gabe, Harley, and Calnan 2015, Petersen et al. 2010). It is also a theme in interviews and focus groups that led us to characterize immunity talk in terms of "choice immunity." In their research on colds and influenza narrative, Prior et al. note that the idea of immunity as a personal possession—"my immunity"—was a prominent theme (2011, page 926). Alongside the biomedical ideas of immunity as a defense against attack from outside and as a method of defining the self in relation to the other was the idea of immunity as acquired, individualized, and a feature of existence over which one had some dominion. A reflexively managed immunity was counterposed with the inevitability of pandemic influenza in a way that intensified the somatic undercurrent of pandemic preparedness and response and set the scene for individualism on matters of pandemic precautions, including vaccination.

Lola, discussed earlier, was again exemplary, but in this instance in connection with the management of immunity:

INTERVIEWER: So did you do anything else around that time to try and avoid catching anything?
LOLA: Oh well we looked after ourselves. We took our preparations that we usually take if we feel we are exposed to something. Like our immune-boosting things. We take Echinacea and vitamin C powder. We usually take that if we've got the slightest signs. We get onto that straight away and take it for two or three days. And nine out of ten times we stop everything. But because this [2009 H1N1] was so prevalent in the community we decided that we'd take the Echinacea daily. I mean not the full dose but we just took some every day as just a little bit of extra [protection].

Lola's account showed that immunity was seen to be open to cultivation since the otherwise standard practice of "immune-boosting" was increased for the case of the 2009 pandemic. This notion of immune boosting is a common trope of advertising and healthcare. Cenovis, which markets vitamins and similar health products, provides consumers with advice on how to promote their immunity (Cenovis 2017). The prestigious Harvard Medical School hosts a website for the general public that has a page devoted to "How to boost your immune system," including advice on diet, exercise, smoking, and stress management (Harvard Medical School 2016). In light of this wide-ranging support for immunity as a consumer and biomedical practice of self, it is not surprising that our respondents made reference to various ways of increasing bodily resilience. It is noteworthy, however, that in response to the appeal to the general public to act in the time of pandemic influenza, Lola and others in our research turned to a consumer-oriented and biomedicalized culture of immunity and its cultivation.

The sense in which immunity culture was implicated in advice to the general public was amplified by the discussion sustained in a Sydney focus group of people in their 40s and without any disclosed vulnerabilities for pandemic influenza. The participants discussed various ways of strengthening the immune system, including chicken soup, in a way that suggested that immunity boosting was a generalized practice necessary for contemporary life:

RACHEL: I mean the herb Echinacea is known to boost the immune system [Yes, it does—that's why I take it] [Yeah] So whenever I've had people that were, clients coming into me saying, "I'm going to India," I'd say, "Well for the first three months before you go, [That's it] take a lot of Echinacea because it builds your system up [Yep] so you can fight it at a higher level." [That's right] And things like elderberry: they're so cheap and easy but they don't dish that out everywhere. [No] And good old chicken soup, you know. Chicken soup's now been scientifically evaluated. They should have soup kitchens at Town Hall.

SABRINA: What for? What's the benefit of chicken soup?

RACHEL: It's got all sorts of health benefits and [Yeah, that's right] restoratives, and strengtheners, and it's . . . You know how it's, it's supposed to—

LISA: Does it depend what you use in the chicken soup though or what sort of chicken it is? Organic chicken or, you know . . . depends where the chicken comes from.

RACHEL: Like for decades, for centuries the, you know, like—

ABBIE: You'll find silverside soup is better than chicken soup.

RACHEL: It's historic. It's in many cultures from Jewish culture and other cultures. Because if something goes wrong, you have chicken soup but it's been like a comfort food. But, in fact, it's now been evaluated. It's the vegetables. The onions . . . Onions are really high in minerals.

SABRINA: Oh yeah, they're good, yeah.

RACHEL: The chicken's really high in calcium [Yeah] because the bones. You put the bones in it for chicken soup [Yeah] you get the bones . . . [Yeah] So if you have a big beef bone, you'd have to use acids to get the bone to disintegrate whereas chicken will do it . . . So chicken or small rabbit ['Cause they're so soft] . . . But yeah, the actual soup's now being analyzed [That's interesting, isn't it?] as a remedy. The herbs you put in: sage is good for flu. You know, like thyme, all those herbs that you use in winter actually have a beneficial effect on the body. [Of course] And so to have that . . . even if you threw sage in the soup and smell it, inhaling it [It's beautiful] is really good for the entire respiratory tract. [That's right]. (Sydney Focus Group, 40s to 60s, No disclosed health problems)

The cultivation of immunity was here attached to tradition and home remedy. These practices connected with wider "care of the body" and through that the contemporary emphasis on self-mastery of one's health and its prospects (Petersen et al. 2010). The cultivation of immunity permitted the subject to act on themselves in light of awareness that the nonpharmaceutical methods—social distancing and hygiene—were unlikely to provide absolute protection. They suggest that immunity was a site for more general preparation of self for life, a perspective that accorded with Emily Martin's account (1994) of immunity practices among United States citizens and its connections with the requirements of the contemporary corporate workplace for resilient and flexible employees. Ed Cohen (2009), too, has remarked on the immunopolitical construction of the contemporary idealized subject of late modern times. Implied, however, in this focus group and across the immunity talk of our respondents was a reassertion of the natural body. Respondents depicted themselves as carefully optimizing the natural capacities of their bodies to cope with infection. Less prominent were biotechnological means, such as antivirals and vaccines.

It is also important to recognize that not everyone we interviewed shared the view that one should be personally active in shaping immunity. In his interview, Rob, from Melbourne and living with HIV, was adamant that infection with influenza was not under volitional control:

INTERVIEWER: So do you think it's inevitable, that, if it's around, you're likely to catch it?
ROB: You're likely to catch it. Yeah. The thing is, some people do, some people don't. It depends on genetics and also it's ... I mean you do all the precautions. Keep, you know, keep clean and that kind of stuff. But I don't think it's gonna have benefit.
[later]
INTERVIEWER: So do you think trying to keep yourself as fit and healthy as possible makes a difference?
ROB: Nup. I think it's a virus. If it wants to get you it will get you. So I think it's just genetics. Wrong place, wrong time. I don't think, everyone's you just can't stop it. If it's gonna get you, it's gonna get you. That's my opinion. (Melbourne, 40s, HIV positive)

In contrast with Rob's view, another of our respondents living with HIV recognized that the modulation of immunity did have relevance for HIV infection, but not, it seemed, for pandemic influenza. Matrix, who was living in Glasgow, spoke of seeking out immune-boosting products to help manage his HIV infection but noted that he had not considered immunity in connection with influenza in general:

> these things are imported from the States. There's a Doctor in San Francisco I think, he's been doing HIV specialist, he's developed this sort of, these sort of vitamins and supplements and stuff. They're quite powerful they're sort of way over the recommended daily allowance . . . so I was assuming that taking very high strength, very potent sort of vitamins and supplements would also help my immune system deal with all these other sort of infections and eh . . . that's what I think. So that's part of my thinking as well but I wouldn't say I had sort of any . . . eh . . . well thought out sort of strategies to deal with other people's flus or colds or sort of chest infections. (Glasgow, 50s, HIV positive)

Matrix's discussion of immune-boosting underlined how, for people with HIV, influenza was a less important infection for them, a theme we pursue in the next chapter. These nuances related to preexisting medical conditions are important to recognize because they reveal considerable diversity with regard to the enactment of the methods for managing influenza infection.

As we have indicated, respondents also spoke of cultivating immunity as a necessary traffic with germs and a related idea that immunity was acquired, most effectively, during childhood, a view that has some scientific support (Olszak et al. 2012). In their joint interview, a Melbourne couple, Anne and Gary, said that exposure to influenza and "dirt" was necessary to build up immunity:

> Anne: Besides, you don't sort of build up any immunity if you never get it [influenza]. I mean it's like these children who are always getting sick 'cause they don't know about dirt 'cause they're not allowed to play in the dirt. I mean you've gotta have some kind of immunity to it. I think we are a bit more careful now because of Gary's lungs than we would have been in the past. I guess the other thing that can lead you to getting something is if you're run down. If there's just too many activities. So I will cut back on things that we've planned to do. (Melbourne, Anne: 60s, No disclosed health problems, Gary: 70s, Chronic illness)

Anne, in her account, spoke for Gary in a manner that suggested the gendering of care in the context of pandemic influenza, since she adopted the care of herself and the more vulnerable Gary. Anne's account foregrounded the idea that exposure to germs—"play in the dirt"—was needed to ensure that bodily immunity was positioned favorably. A related idea was that the body's vitality could be dispersed easily through overexertion. Anne's account also exposed the tension between the need to protect Gary due to his vulnerability and the idea that immunity depended on connections with others.

Like Anne, Gordon, whose narrative we explored in the previous chapter, outlined at length the orthodox influenza avoidance measures encouraged by health authorities. But he counterpointed these strategies with the necessity of "germs":

GORDON: I'm not a great advocate of all these antibacterial washes and things like that. I just think that they also kill the good germs as well. You know? And our bodies are very adaptable. We get things once and we suffer through for a couple of weeks but then we brought up our own anti—whatever it is we build up—and we don't get it again, usually. It's usually only one-off, a lot of these things because our bodies adjust and so I don't think we need to kill off everything, all the germs we've got because some of the germs are so good. And you've only gotta look at the kids. I look at my grandkids and I think they live in a sterile society. I never did, you know. Well I didn't. I don't know about you but I never did. I was always covered in dirt and something, you know. I mean I've led a fairly healthy life. I'm still here! I'm still here.

INTERVIEWER: Absolutely. So is that a sense of building up immunity in some way?

GORDON: It's important. I think it's important. It's important. You see ads now for everything, it's so sterile. Everything is sterile. You've gotta have germs. Gotta have germs. That's how your body builds up against them. (Melbourne, 60s, Lung disease)

In this view, immunity was built up during childhood and was therefore a feature of physical maturation. Implied too was a notion of the body's immunity as educable. This view does cohere with scientific accounts of immunity that suggest that important milestones in the development of individual immunity are reached during childhood (Jenhalm 2011, Marques et al. 2013). There is a literature, too, which has explored the development of immunity in the fetus during pregnancy and therefore of the complex and as yet not fully understood process of the immune response in pregnant women (Holt and Jones 2000, Ygberg and Nilsson 2012).

Gordon's account also drew out the paradoxical way in which immunity was understood as a defense of the body and that immunity was developed only through commune with potential pathogens. This paradox revealed how self/not self immunity and network immunity were combined in talk on immunity. Gordon's account also rejected the immunity culture of the contemporary consumer, harking back nostalgically to his own past when playing with dirt had strengthened his ability to survive microbial threat to life. This account therefore mobilized a canonical narrative of nature versus culture and more specifically the naturalistic communion of the developing immune system with the microbial life found in dirt versus the artificial and, apparently, unhealthy sterility of the present. Gordon specifically noted how contemporary advertising did injury to this naturalistic dimension of immunity.

Gordon's account echoed the *War of the Worlds* narrative where alien life was in the end defeated, not by human effort, but by nature. This recourse to nature is another way in which pandemic influenza threw individuals back on themselves, in this instance into their past and their relationship with natural exposures to immunity-building pathogens. It also resonated with the observations we have made regarding the weak enactment of social distancing advocated by public health, as discussed in chapter 4. A pandemic influenza event is such that it cannot be avoided, despite the of best intentions, so subjects are forced into a retreat from biomedical technologies and back into their relationships with their bodies and, in turn, their embodied relation with nature.

Other interviewees shared Gordon's nostalgia for the natural methods of resisting pathogens. In this interview extract, Alex, with chronic lung disease, concurred with the idea that parents should be responsible for their children's immunity and made the point that this was particularly the case since, apparently, the immune system was formed in childhood:

INTERVIEWER: Do you like carry sanitizer around with you, things like that?
ALEX: No. Actually, for someone who's got lung disease, I'm, not really much of a germ-a-phobe. I know it contradicts what I just said, but I'm much more of a believer, particularly with children that, if I ever have children, that kids should be exposed to mud, a bit of mud, a bit of muck, but of

all this sort of stuff because, in their early years, because that's when they build their immune system. So I'm not actually a person who obsessively washes their hands or anything like that. (Sydney, 30s, Lung disease)

Alex showed an interest, then, in figuring herself in particular ways, indicating social expectations (even moral constraints) concerning the reflexive management of immunity. Through reference to "germ-a-phobe" her account echoed, too, Mitzi's use of "germ freak," discussed earlier. Both Alex and Mitzi shared the status of someone with a preexisting lung disease that predisposed them to potentially severe illness in the case of pandemic influenza. But both were concerned to manage this risk in ways that did not jeopardize relationships with others and their social standing. Suggested here, then, was that the management of immunity raised questions of identity—of who one is and is not—most obviously in relation to self-care. For Alex, however, there was an added layer of complexity since she spoke of her parental responsibility to "educate" the immune systems of her children by exposing them to "a bit if muck" in tensions with her own status as someone who believed she should take precautions.

Other respondents made it clear that the management of one's immunity came with social expectations. In this lengthy extract from a focus group of 20-something healthy adults in Melbourne, the respondents reflected on "immunity training" through exposure to dirt as already noted. But in addition they spoke favorably of parents who had provided these opportunities:

SALLY: My parents thoroughly encouraged playing in the dirt and getting into like all the . . . like playing with all the animals and stuff. Just getting in there, really. And I think it does, actually, if you get in there young and end up getting exposed to all those germs. [I think you pick them up] Yeah.
INTERVIEWER: So do you think that does build up immunity? [Mmm]
MELANIE: I think getting sick every so often is a good thing 'cause it builds your immune system up. So, so if you do get something really nasty, hopefully that helps.
INTERVIEWER: So how do you feel about that?
MELANIE: Until I started high school I was really, really healthy; there was virtually nothing wrong with me. I don't, I think I only had one day off school when I was at primary school. It was, I don't know, I just, we did whatever we wanted and mum didn't really stop us from doing things. If we got dirty that was that.

JOSH: You eat a lot of mud as a kid. I think it's part of growing up.
MELANIE: Especially boys.
JOSH: Yeah. See I was a younger brother. You were the older brother. So you would have definitely eaten a bit of mud.
MELANIE: He would have fed you mud. We, yeah, look we, we had all sorts of things going around in our family.
JOSH: Yeah. I'm sure I ate a fair bit of dirt. "Eat this Josh." And I was never, I was never frightened in the backyard and getting dirty.
MELANIE: Yeah, my sister did too. [Really?]
SALLY: We used to dig down past the dirt to the clay so you could make pots and stuff. [Oh yeah]
JOSH: Yeah. I remember doing that. I planned to build a house once.
INTERVIEWER: How far did you get?
JOSH: I built one, one brick out of mud but that was about it, yeah. Lost interest.
INTERVIEWER: So you had the sense of by being out, being exposed to all those things that it actually helps you?
JOSH: Yeah. I mean I've got no science behind it. It's just I guess a personal opinion.
MELANIE: I don't think shielding kids from that is necessarily a good thing. You know, either from the perspective of letting them get, you know, in contact with germs and stuff like that but also just from being a kid and restricting a child from what they wanna do. There's obviously limits but, you know, it feels a bit, yeah, it doesn't, doesn't feel right, doesn't feel right.
INTERVIEWER: To stop them?
MELANIE: To stop kids from doing just what you do and getting dirty, playing in the mud, all that sort of stuff.
INTERVIEWER: How do you feel about that?
OSCAR: Yeah. I think it's better for the immune system if you're a bit close to germs. (Melbourne Focus Group, 20s, No disclosed health problems)

In this focus group, "mud" was the sign for pathogens that stimulated immune responses. But "mud" also connoted other meanings, such as nature, matter out of place, transgressive blurring of boundaries, taking risks as a matter of learning about the self and the world, and the implied learning and discovery associated with childhood play. The narrative sustained by these young people also suggested that the cultivation of immunity during childhood was not only a practical matter of strengthening the ability of the body to survive pathogens, it also concerned an orientation to the future of the self which had the proportions of how to "be-in-the-world" and its uncertainties (Giddens 1991). Immunity in this sense was a mode of reflexive self-care imbued with biological, biographical, and ontological importance. The cultivation of immunity, then, was figured as a matter of the choices one makes and of the choices parents made for the younger self, suggesting reflexive modernization and the notion of the choice "biography" and its imperatives and anxieties (Beck and Beck-Gernsheim 2002).

Missing in the talk on choice immunity, however, was reference to collective immunity and the protection of vulnerable people. Omission of talk on altruistic management of immunity raised the prospect that contemporary immunopolitics are individualized and have therefore abandoned the collective mobilization of public life in relation to pandemic threat. Politically and biologically, immunity is foremost a method of signifying how self is distinguished from other in the process of detecting and destroying pathogens. The previous examples have shown how our respondents used this construction of immunity to talk about how they focussed on the interior body and to strengthen it in the face of pandemic influenza. The bubble metaphor used by people with lung disease and its echoes in the accounts of others signaled that absolute protection was understood to require a kind of separation from social life that was untenable and undesirable. As the accounts we have discussed in this and the previous two chapters have revealed, the focus on self mobilized the idea of oneself as "at risk" but less talk on oneself as "a risk." Those with lung disease were aware that others presented a risk to them, at times with some consternation that people failed to use social distance and hygiene measures. Respondents spoke of local agreements between themselves and family and friends to avoid each other while ill and Cameron, from chapter 1, assumed he was infected and tried to avoid contact with family members. But for the most part, people in our research spoke very little of the idea that they may present a risk to others. Absent was the idea that social distancing, hygiene, antivirals, and vaccination were technologies available to our respondents for them to inhibit the spread of infection to others and therefore help to manage the pandemic in a collective sense and serve to protect the vulnerable. This absence was most obvious in connection with vaccination. Influenza vaccination, as it was in 2009, was targeted toward the vulnerable to protect them from infection. But vaccination is also a way of controlling the spread of a virus in a population. For pandemic influenza, vaccination of healthcare workers, particularly those who provide care for vulnerable patients, was regarded as a way of reducing the risk of transmission to the vulnerable. Childhood vaccination, for example, is regarded as a way of inhibiting the circulation of pathogens in populations, commonly referred to as "herd" immunity (Quadri-Sheriff et al. 2012).

This lack of discussion of protecting others is traceable into the orthodox view of immunity as a biological mechanism of recognition of self in distinction to other and of the other as alien to self. As noted, this is a view of self that is supported by the long-standing notion of immunity as a suspension of duty to the other for the sake of self-interest. As Cohen has delineated (2009), immunity is a political concept that gave Koch and other biomedical scientists a metaphor for their discovery of the action of cells on pathogens coming into the body. The "discovery" of biomedical immunity can be thought of as an important moment in the constitution of the somatic, individualized self, defined against the other. As our respondents indicated, immunity has retained the double meaning of biological regime of truth and politics of self-definition, but in ways that may undercut acting for the good of the other. It is important to recognize this effect of immunity talk since it foregrounds embodied and individualized choice and obscures collective action. As we also indicated, the turn to the fabrication of bodily resilience involved a turn to naturalism in matters of health and by implication, away from biotechnology. These currents in immunological subjective life are perhaps reflected in the weak uptake of hygiene, social distancing, and vaccines. We have shown, then, how the pandemic story, wedded as it is to particular forms of immunopolitics, constitutes problems for itself. Our respondents did act for others in some circumstances, particularly parents and carers of those with specific vulnerabilities, but it also seemed to be the case that such action did not have the sanctions enjoyed by individualized forms of self-care. It is reasonable to ask what other narratives on pandemics and immunity might possibly enlarge how publics can act for themselves and others in productive ways?

References

Beck, U, and E Beck-Gernsheim. 2002. *Individualisation: Institutionalised individualism and its social and political consequences.* London: Sage.

Briggs, C, and M Nichter. 2009. "Biocommunicability and the biopolitics of pandemic threats." *Medical Anthropology* 28 (3):189–198.

Burges Watson, D, T Moreira, and M Murtagh. 2009. "Little bottles and the promise of probiotics." *Health* 13 (2):219–234. doi: 10.1177/1363459308099685.

CDC. 2014. "How flu spreads." Accessed May 1, 2017. http://www.cdc.gov/flu/about/disease/spread.htm.
Cenovis. 2017. "All you need to know about boosting your immune system." Accessed May 1, 2017. http://cenovis.com.au/how-to-boost-your-immune-system/.
Cohen, E. 2009. *A body worth defending: Immunity, biopolitics and the apotheosis of the modern body*. Durham and London: Duke University Press.
Davis, M, P Flowers, D Lohm, E Waller, and N Stephenson. 2016. "Immunity, biopolitics and pandemics: Public and individual responses to the threat to life." *Body & Society* 22 (4):130–154.
Dettol. 2013. "Dettol mission for health: The strength of a single mum—See Nicole's story." Accessed May 1, 2017. https://www.youtube.com/watch?v=Si89gX6YVrE.
Foucault, M. 2007. *Security, territory, population: Lectures at the College de France, 1977-1978*. New York: Picador.
Gabe, J, K Harley, and M Calnan. 2015. "Healthcare choice: Discourse, perceptions, experiences and practices." *Current Sociology Monograph* 63 (5):623–635.
Gerlach, N, and S Hamilton. 2014. "Trafficking in the zombie: The CDC Zombie Apocalypse campaign, diseaseability and pandemic culture." *Refractory: A Journal of Entertainment Media*, June 24. http://refractory.unimelb.edu.au/2014/06/26/cdc-zombie-apocalypse-gerlach-hamilton/.
Giddens, A. 1991. *Modernity and self identity: Self and society in the late modern age*. London: Polity.
Haraway, D. 1999. "The biopolitics of postmodern bodies: Determinations of self in immune system discourse." In *Feminist theory and the body: A reader*, edited by J Price and M Shildrick, 203–214. Edinburgh: Edinburgh University Press.
Harvard Medical School. 2016. "How to boost your immune system." Accessed May 1, 2017. http://www.health.harvard.edu/staying-healthy/how-to-boost-your-immune-system.
Holt, P, and C Jones. 2000. "The development of the immune system during pregnancy and early life." *Allergy* 55:688–697.
Honigsbaum, M. 2013. "Regulating the 1918–19 pandemic: Flu, stoicism and the Northcliffe Press." *Medical History* 57 (2):165–185. doi: http://dx.doi.org/10.1017/mdh.2012.101.
Jamieson, M. 2015. "The politics of immunity: Reading Cohen through Canguilheim and new materialism." *Body & Society* 22 (4):106–129.
Jenhalm, M. 2011. "Childhood immune maturation and allergy development: Regulation by maternal immunity and microbial exposure." *American Journal of Reproductive Immunology* 66 (Suppl 1):75–80.
Kleiser, R. 1976. *The boy in the plastic bubble*. United States: TV Movie.
Koteyko, N. 2009. "'I am a very happy, lucky lady, and I am full of vitality!' Analysis of promotional strategies on the websites of probiotic yoghurt producers." *Critical Discourse Studies* 6 (2):111–125.
Lundgren, B. 2015. "The common cold, influenza and immunity in post-pandemic times: Lay representations of self and Other among older people in Sweden." *Health, Culture and Society* 8 (2):ISSN 2161-6590 (online). doi 10.5195/hcs.2015.200.
Marques, A, T O'Connor, C Roth, E Susser, and A Bjorke-Monsen. 2013. "The influence of maternal prenatal and early childhood nutrition and maternal prenatal stress on offspring immune system development and neurodevelopmental disorders." *Frontiers in Neuroscience* 7:120.
Martin, A. 2010. "Microchimerism in the Mother(land): Blurring the borders of body and nation." *Body & Society* 16 (3):23–50.

Martin, E. 1994. *Flexible bodies: Tracking immunity in American culture from the days of polio to the age of AIDS*. Boston: Beacon Press.

Mitchell, T, DL Dee, CR Phares, et al. 2011. "Non-pharmaceutical interventions during an outbreak of 2009 pandemic influenza A (H1N1) virus infection at a large public university, April–May 2009." *Clinical Infectious Diseases* 52 (Suppl 1):S138–S145.

Nasiruddin, M, M Halabi, A Dao, K Chen, and B Brown. 2013. "Zombies—A pop culture resource for public health awareness." *Emerging Infectious Diseases* 19:809+.

Nerlich, B, and N Koteyko. 2008. "Balancing food risks and food benefits: The coverage of probiotics in the UK national press." *Sociological Research Online* 13 (3):1.

Olszak, T, D An, S Zeissig, M Vera, J Richter, A Franke, J Glickman, R Siebert, R Baron, D Kasper, and R Blumberg. 2012. "Microbial exposure during early life has persistent effects on natural killer T cell function." *Science* 336 (27 April):489–493.

Pelling, M. 1997. "Contagion/germ theory/specificity." In *Companion encyclopedia of the history of medicine*, edited by W Bynum and R Porter, 309–334. Abingdon: Routledge.

Petersen, A, M Davis, S Fraser, and J Lindsay. 2010. "Healthy living and citizenship: An overview." *Critical Public Health* 20 (4):391–400.

Petryna, A 2003. *Life exposed: Biological citizens after Chernobyl*. Princeton: Princeton University Press.

Prior, L, M Evans, and H Prout. 2011. "Talking about colds and flu: The lay diagnosis of two common illnesses among older British people." *Social Science & Medicine* 73:922–928.

Quadri-Sheriff, M, K Hendrix, S Downs, L Sturm, G Zimet, and S Finnell. 2012. "The role of herd immunity in parents' decision to vaccinate children: A systematic review." *Pediatrics* 130 (3):1.

Rose, N, and C Novas. 2005. "Biological citizenship." In *Global assemblages: Technology, politics, and ethics as anthropological problems*, edited by A Ong and S Collier, 439–463. Malden, MA: Blackwell.

Rubin, G, R Amlot, L Page, and S Wessely. 2009. "Public perceptions, anxiety, and behaviour change in relation to the swine flu outbreak: Cross sectional telephone survey." *British Medical Journal* 339:b2651.

Seale, H, M McLaws, A Heywood, K Ward, C Lowbridge, D Van, J Gralton, and C MacIntyre. 2009. "The community's attitude towards swine flu and pandemic influenza." *Medical Journal of Australia* 191 (5):267–269.

Wald, P. 2008. *Contagious: Cultures, carriers, and the outbreak narrative*. Durham: Duke University Press.

Ygberg, S, and A Nilsson. 2012. "The developing immune system—from foetus to toddler." *Acta Paediatrica* 101:120–127.

6
Vulnerabilities

> As an African woman, I'm not scared of the flu because I've seen something bigger than swine flu. I've seen something bigger like HIV where I saw people very close to me dying slowly over a period of years . . . there was no medication, there was nothing. So I think swine flu, where I'm sitting, doesn't really scare me. (Heather, Glasgow, 40s, Focus group with Black African women with HIV)

> People don't understand that yes I might look healthy but I'm not, and I could be really unhealthy if I got this flu. It's quite difficult to get people to understand . . . yeah. It's really hard to explain to people that just because I look healthy doesn't mean I am. (Marlene, Sydney, 30s, Lung disease)

In the previous chapters we have explored the importance of contagion and immunity for public responses to the pandemic. In this chapter, we consider the identity positions that pertained to public health advice and related questions of agency and constraint. As noted previously, pandemic communications in 2009 and since have made explicit reference to two identities: a generalized healthy citizen who is asked to prepare themselves for the possibility of a public health emergency, and a vulnerable citizen who, due to preexisting biomedical and social conditions, is more likely to experience morbidity and mortality related to viral outbreak. In the United Kingdom, for example, messages on pandemic preparedness and advice regarding vaccines were given to the general population and to those seen as more likely to experience severe disease (Hine 2010). A similar hierarchy of the healthy and the vulnerable was used in Australia (Australian Government Department of Health and Ageing 2011). This tiered approach of health and vulnerability reflected a biomedical conceptualization of risk used to ration and focus resources. Our research explored these subject positions in light of real-world contexts and

Pandemics, Publics, and Narrative. Mark Davis and Davina Lohm, Oxford University Press (2020).
© Oxford University Press.
DOI: 10.1093/oso/9780190683764.001.0001

the temporalized, unfolding character of the pandemic and related social and biographical considerations of preexisting health status and, for some women, the coincident advent of pregnancy. As we will see, pandemic subjects are complexly and troublingly positioned in pandemic time, biography, and other social aspects of their engagements with microbial threat.

Pandemic experience can be conceptualized as in part an intersection of history (the pandemic event) and biography (one's life circumstances). This confluence of history and biography is perhaps most strident in the policy configurations of vulnerability that come into being in the time of a severe outbreak. The United Kingdom identified as vulnerable groups people with severe respiratory illness, preexisting illness, pregnant women, and children under three years of age (Department of Health United Kingdom 2007). Australian plans identified the same groups (Australian Department of Health and Ageing 2008) but also included the very elderly and those with immune dysfunction associated with cancer or HIV. With the advent of the 2009 pandemic, Australia also identified Indigenous people as at risk, and strategies were tailored specifically for them (Australian Government Department of Health and Ageing 2011). These vulnerability categories, as we have seen, were reflected in news and health communications. For example, an Australian Broadcasting Corporation television news item from July 16, 2009, reported on the rise of the pandemic in Australia and pregnant women (ABC News NSW 2009): "The latest group being cautioned to take particular care is pregnant women." The reporter went on to make reference to the pandemic preparedness message and the plight of some hospitalized pregnant women: "The message has a familiar ring: don't be alarmed, just alert. Six pregnant women in Sydney have recently been put on life support with swine flu." This news item identified pregnant women as a group at heightened risk and combined it with the "Be alert, not alarmed" advice we discussed in chapter 3. The naming and explanation of vulnerability was therefore a feature of public life during 2009, made visible in the images used to construct television news and other multimedia offerings.

Vulnerability categories like "pregnant women," however, fix what we want to argue are more dynamic forms of coming into being of identities and practices in connection with a pandemic and the characteristics of one's biomedical situation and life world. We used these vulnerability identity categories to organize our own research, and they inform this chapter, but we want to "unfreeze" these identities to reveal more of how lives are lived in the time of pandemic. We assume that personal experience narrative is a window on how history and biography are negotiated in general and in the particular case of pandemic influenza. The stories we tell reflect how we contend with the conditions of possibility we encounter, as narratives on surviving illness (Frank 1995) and the broken narratives of people with disability (Hyden and Brockmeier 2008), are said to do. Stories of vulnerability, therefore, reveal how these categories were made meaningful, appropriated, nuanced, or resisted by those addressed by public health messages. A particular focus for us is also how narrators choose to make their so-called vulnerability visible to others and for what purposes.

Another consideration is that the categories of vulnerability that inform public policy are largely based on a priori notions of pandemic risk and its management, but they gloss over important contextual features of lived experience. Pandemic policymaking can be construed as medicalizing; that is, it defines social life in medical terms, "to make medical," as Peter Conrad has put it (2013, page 196). Contemporary public health systems are generally understood to emphasize a relatively autonomous subject who is willing and able to take up their own healthcare as a matter of choice biography (Petersen et al. 2010). The subject is said to be individualized and to engage in the commodification of health and healthcare, to focus on their health as a personal possession and their bodies as the basis for the production of healthy, biological selfhood (Rose 2007). Vulnerability categories—people with preexisting medical conditions, particularly those involving respiratory and or immune function, the very elderly, and pregnant women—are highly medicalized identity labels that gloss over questions of autonomy, context, and individualized self-commodification, both between and within vulnerability categories. For example, in their review of research on the structural determinants of responses to pandemic communications, Lin et al. (2014) identified how social characteristics such as age, gender, education, and media consumption preferences shaped knowledge of pandemics and reported compliance with guidelines. As we will show, considerable nuance is in evidence in the narrative accounts provided by people who participated in our research. Pregnant women were only gradually persuaded into their "at risk" status, while others, such as people with HIV, found pandemic risk identity to be less relevant than what they regarded to be the more pressing ones of aging and HIV or living as black African mothers with HIV in the United Kingdom. Gender, and specifically the gendering of action taken to address pandemic influenza, is implied in different forms of vulnerability and in different ways, for example, in the case of pregnant women at greater risk but also in families and couples where one person, typically a woman according to our respondents, provided care for others. As we will explore, too, people with lung disease and those with HIV were already living highly medicalized lives at the time of the 2009 pandemic and spoke of how they readily took up the technologies and dispositions advocated for in the response to pandemic influenza. This double medicalization is another way in which differences are complexly articulated with pandemic influenza.

In addition, the earlier quotations from Heather and Marlene draw attention to how they, in different ways, positioned themselves (Davies and Harre 1990) in their narrative reflections on vulnerability. Heather made pandemic influenza less of a problem than her HIV infection and set the pandemic into the context of her life as an asylum seeker and the more general situation for her life and health in Africa compared with Scotland. Heather, therefore, pointed out that the pandemic comes into health contexts that transform its meanings and appraisal of its threats. In this view, the biopolitical rationalities of HIV citizenship are necessarily articulated with those of pandemic influenza and, as Heather suggests, myriad other challenges including national citizenship in the form of residency in the United Kingdom. Marlene spoke of her invisibility to others as "at risk," a situation that appeared to make the negotiation of precautions difficult. These accounts of responses to pandemic risk can also be understood through the lens of intersectionality, which draws attention to the ways that, for example, gender identity, life history, biomedical situation, and interpersonal life combine in lived experience and condition the possibilities for individual and collective agency (Hankivsky 2012). Building on Heather's comments, in what follows we investigate the complexities of vulnerability in light of preexisting health conditions but also through the lenses of the age and generation nexus, the gendering of action on pandemic risk, and pregnancy. We also pick up on Marlene's account of health identity to explore how people "at risk" for pandemic influenza disclosed this information, shaped relations with others, and therefore negotiated for the cooperation of people who might pose "a risk" to the vulnerable.

(In)vulnerabilities

In previous chapters we have indicated that those deemed to be vulnerable and those with multiple risks, for example, pregnant women with lung disease, had become acutely aware of their risk status during the 2009 pandemic. The young and healthy, in contrast, appeared to take the position of the invulnerable, assuming that influenza would not be a consequential health experience for them, even if they were infected. These perspectives concurred with the focus groups conducted in Scotland by Hilton and Smith (2010), who found that those most at risk appeared to be most concerned and voluble on the pandemic and its implications for health. This separation among our respondents according to their relative (in)vulnerability can be construed as an effect of medicalization (Conrad 2013, page 196) or, in other terms, the application of medical rationality to the construction of risk identities. Those who came to recognize themselves as at heightened risk had also taken on pandemic discourse as a technology of self (Rose 2007), marking themselves as biological citizens of pandemic time but also finding themselves separated from others. The narratives offered by our participants also show that vulnerability and its alterity, invulnerability, were both considerably nuanced by other social factors of age and generation, gender, pregnancy, and preexisting medical conditions.

Old Timers' Disease

Younger and older respondents appeared to have had different viewpoints on the advent of the pandemic, partly due to a sense of invulnerability that younger people appropriated and because older people had experienced more health events in their lives, including previous pandemics. In this extract from her interview, Brigitte, introduced in chapter 4, commented on the pandemic as a risk for younger and older, vulnerable people and therefore not necessarily herself:

INTERVIEWER: So I suppose the next thing is: can you tell me what a pandemic flu is as opposed to just sort of normal flu? Do you know what's the difference?
BRIGITTE: Well from what I'm hearing in the news and things like that it's just a flu that would cause death to people who are vulnerable. Children or elderly people. And it obviously wipes out a lot of people catching it.
INTERVIEWER: So what sorts of things have you heard about the flu, particularly the pandemic?
BRIGITTE: Things like bird flu which perhaps originated in Asia. And then could have been, could be brought over. People were kept in isolation in

Singapore, places like that. And then some healthcare practitioners died from it and things like that because of exposure. People will be isolated, it's quite a serious thing. And it was taken seriously and people were inoculated. And also that the people that are affected are more likely to be people with a preexisting condition. Someone who's older, you know. Their immunity might not be so great. (Melbourne, 40s, No disclosed health problems)

Brigitte appeared to conflate pandemic influenza with avian influenza in her interview, signaling how her engagement with the 2009 pandemic was rather generalized. Brigitte's account did, however, refer to pandemic communications in Australia from May 2009 that reinforced the advice that vulnerable people were more at risk of serious complications. Implied in Brigitte's account was the idea that other vulnerable people were affected and therefore she was not. This way of accounting for vulnerability implied a normative, not old, not young, healthy self as the flip-side of vulnerability.

Time, age, and generation were implicated in narrative on pandemic influenza in other ways that accentuated a sense of personal invulnerability. In a Melbourne interview, Chris, aged in his 20s and from the healthy group, likened influenza to an "old timers'" disease from the 1800s Gold Rush in Australia:

INTERVIEWER: Now you couldn't remember whether you'd had the flu vaccine or not.
CHRIS: No.
INTERVIEWER: Okay. Maybe you just want to talk through why you think that you can't remember?
CHRIS: Well I mean I remember in primary school and high school just lining up for specific needles and vaccines. And sort of go with the flow because you got a free lolly or something like that. I didn't really pay attention to what it was. Or I did at the time but I quickly forgot. I don't know. You sort of think, when I think of influenza, I sort of think of the Gold Rush like with Ballarat [city at the center of the gold rush in Victoria] and stuff, because I think a lot of people died of influenza there under those conditions. And you sort of think of it as like an old timers' disease ... so maybe I was vaccinated against it at an early age and then I just stopped caring about it.

INTERVIEWER: So you don't really associate flu or dangerous flu with our time?

CHRIS: Well when I get a cough or a cold, or anything, I sort of just ignore it. I have to be pushed to go to the doctor's or anything to get it fixed. I sort of just wait for it to pass out because you think it's just one of those things that's going around. You just take it as it is really. (Melbourne, 20s, No disclosed health problems)

Influenza was in this account temporalized in two ways: set back in time; and associated with the aged. Chris's account showed how time can also be a form of protective distance, echoing chapter 4, which considered the metaphorical connotations of social distance. Like many of the younger, healthy people in our research, Chris appeared to take his health for granted and thought of influenza as not a risk for himself. As noted, pandemic communications emphasized that some groups were at heightened risk, a message that may have mobilized an implicit invulnerability and given those who identified as healthy a message that the infection would not be a problem for them. Chris's account also indicated a narrative of medical triumph over disease, supported by a view of the pandemic as a health problem for a previous era of healthcare. The idea that the pandemic was a Gold Rush disease underlined the idea that modern medicine had transcended the threat posed by pandemic influenza.

Living in a time of biomedical advancement was also a comforting factor for Natalie, who participated in a Melbourne focus group with other women and men from the healthy group. She was aware of the treatments available if she became unwell and was sufficiently confident in them to not worry:

And I guess the bit I wasn't so worried about is that they did really have things to treat it with. If you caught it, if you understood it early enough, there were treatments available. And I guess that gave me . . . If I knew if I caught it and I'd die, I'm sure I'd be a lot more worried about it. But considering there was Tamiflu, I was fine. I was, "Oh well, I should be right." (Melbourne Focus Group, 20s, No disclosed health problems)

For Natalie and Chris, above, living with twenty-first-century medicine was seen to provide the necessary treatments for influenza. The benefits of contemporary medicine were also apparent to older people in our research who recalled times when infectious diseases were more significant problems. When speaking about her past experience of epidemics, Roslyn made reference to polio vaccination and the transformation of health expectations with which it was associated:

ROSLYN: You don't get sort of epidemic measles and chicken pox anymore and polio's sort of gone now and all that sort of stuff.
INTERVIEWER: So you haven't had any experiences say with polio?
ROSLYN: Not too much, no. Because the vaccine was coming into being when I was a child. And my mother's friend, her son contracted polio. He was not vaccinated. And he contracted it. And it sort of made everybody think that this is something that you really, if its available, you take it.
INTERVIEWER: Right. So were you already vaccinated before then?
ROSLYN: Yes. We were the very first people to have the vaccine in our area, in England. Yes. So we were sort of the guinea pigs so to speak. But it seems to have worked.
INTERVIEWER: So there was a response from the community when he got it? Were more people inclined to be vaccinated?
ROSLYN: Yes there was. Yeah. And it was all shock, horror! Really all shock, horror! Because both my parents had polio as children and survived without any sort of major problems. Luckily, 'cause there was a lot of problems resulting from polio. Both mum and dad knew the consequences. (Melbourne, 60s, No disclosed health problems)

Roslyn's story of polio marked a generational change in the management of infectious diseases that benefited her and, in turn, Chris and Natalie. This reference to generational change is another important temporal organization of pandemic narrative that informed how people in our research spoke of pandemic influenza. Another reference to polio emerged in an interview with Katrina, who was living in Melbourne and in her 70s. Like Roslyn, Katrina linked polio with fear and referred to a period when avoiding infection was the only available public health strategy:

I s'pose when I was a child polio was an epidemic and suddenly we were just terrified. It was before immunization. Before all that sort of stuff. And all I can remember from that is being very frightened and there were all the things you weren't supposed to do. You weren't supposed to go to the pictures.

You weren't supposed to be in a crowd. You weren't supposed to swim in the swimming pool. You weren't supposed to, at one stage, eat ice cream. And I was with a friend one day and he ate ice cream. It was so terrible.... Oh the guilt and the fear; it was terrible. My brother did, my youngest brother got polio but a lot later. Basically, they didn't want anyone with it. It did hurt. So that was very frightening. And my generation we all had measles, mumps, chicken pox, you name it. (Melbourne, 70s, Older group)

Katrina's memories of fear and guilt associated with polio and other infectious diseases of childhood gave the impression of a period in medical history that contrasted starkly with the taken-for-granted confidence in contemporary public health depicted by Chris and Natalie. Margaret also from Melbourne and in her 70s, had clear memories of previous influenza infections:

INTERVIEWER: Have you had the flu?
MARGARET: Yes, I have had it. I had it, I think it must, it was in 1957. It was just before I was married. I remember that; it made a vivid impression. I think that might have been the first lot of Asian flu that ever came to Australia and that was nasty. And then I had another bout of it sometime in the seventies. I can't quite remember when. I always seem to manage to do these things in the school holidays.
[later]
I had another bout of it in 2003 and that was not long after my husband died. And he'd been very ill for a fair while. And I was very run-down. And I ended up in hospital at that time with pneumonia. So ... but they're the only three times I can remember because you don't forget when you've had the flu, really. It's nasty, isn't it? (Melbourne, 70s, Older group)

Margaret remembered her illnesses with influenza and they seemed to have been associated with important milestones in her life. The 1957 influenza to which Margaret referred may have been the 1957–1958 pandemic that was first observed in Hong Kong (Kilbourne 2006). Roslyn, Katrina, and Margaret appeared able to recall lifetimes where infectious diseases had been realities. Chris and Natalie appeared to have had no such recollections, perhaps a reflection of their younger age and their membership of a generation that lives after vaccine technologies.

Man Flu

Our research also showed that gender relations were implicated in the healthcare labor required in time of pandemic influenza. Pippa, aged in her 30s and living in Sydney with lung disease, provided an account of her role in the management of pandemic influenza and her relationship with her partner:

INTERVIEWER: Do you make your husband get a vaccine as well for the flu?
PIPPA: Yes, I do, the poor man. I think he does it, yeah, he does it 'cause I strongly request him to. I think he's indulging me.
INTERVIEWER: Does he take any other measures as well? Does he keep a bottle of sanitizer?
PIPPA: No he doesn't and I encourage him to. When swine flu happened, because he's catching the bus home from work, I was making him. (Sydney, 30s, Lung disease)

Pippa situated vaccination and hygiene in her relationship and her health status and made links with gender identity in healthcare. The phrases "indulging me" and "I was making him," indicated that Pippa tried to shape the behavior of her partner and that he was somewhat resistant. Public health communications predominantly appeal to the atomized individual. Pippa's account indicated that pandemic communications mobilize not just individuals but also the gendered intersubjective relations of partnerships in the domestic sphere. It is likely, then, that communications on pandemic threat address women who perform healthcare for their partners, children, and the elderly. These gendered dynamics of pandemic and seasonal influenza care may explain why surveys find that women are more likely to report that they comply with public health advice than are men, as Lin et al. noted (2014). Pippa's narrative and others like it in our research suggest how gendered relations mediate how publics enact the advice of public health authorities, a feature of the public response that is not commonly discussed in pandemic preparedness and response plans.

We also found that the diversity of family life was important to the work of women as mothers and health carers. Claire, first discussed in chapter 4, reflected on the health status of her ex-partner, his risk of pandemic influenza and the health of her children. She depicted herself as the central figure in the management of these considerations:

CLAIRE: I think as well, like, their [her children's] dad is quite vulnerable and he gets the flu jab, but my kids are not entitled to it. So it's like (laughs) you're trying to protect, but you're not following it through because kids carry it quite a lot and they have contact with their dad but they don't get the flu jab.

INTERVIEWER: And how does that situation make you feel?

CLAIRE: (sigh) I was a bit annoyed when I phoned the GP to ask if they [Claire's children] could get it, I was just told, "No," and even when I explained why I was asking they just said because the kids didn't have any underlying health issues they're not entitled to it. But I was saying, "Yeah, but their parents do." So everybody could pass it onto their dad and that could potentially knock him out you know what I mean (laughs) and they have a lot of contact so to me it would make more sense to immunize the whole family. But then I'm a bit worried about what they're putting into my kids! (laughs) So it's so hard to know what to do.

INTERVIEWER: So you did say this to the GP?

CLAIRE: I asked the GP to immunize the kids, if they could get the flu jab because the parents get it because of their father, yeah, and they said no.

INTERVIEWER: No? Even though you said why?

CLAIRE: Yeah.

INTERVIEWER: And was this this year [2012]?

CLAIRE: Yeah. And I'm not entitled to it either, I was entitled to it when it was swine flu because I was pregnant but I'm not entitled to the annual flu jab.

[later]

INTERVIEWER: Is this something that you'd talked about with the children's dad?

CLAIRE: Not really (laughs). It's something that I kind of take on myself because I don't want to scare them and I don't want their dad to feel I'm making a big issue out of his health, so it's just a strange situation. (laughs) But I also have a lot of friends that are really vulnerable and I get paranoid if I've got a cough or and I don't want to see them. It's quite difficult because on one hand you feel like making an issue if that person has got a condition and you're worried about that but on the other hand you don't want to make it embarrassing for them. "Oh I've got a cough I can't come near you in case I kill you!" (laughs) You know what I mean? (Glasgow, 30s, Pregnant in 2009)

In this small story of Claire's engagement with the management of health, the responsible mother and friend was depicted as having to take on the public health system, but not with complete satisfaction. Notably, Claire took on the health vulnerability of her children's father as a matter for her to consider, reinforcing the argument that healthcare in relation to pandemic influenza is relational and feminized. These gendered responsibilities appeared to have persisted in Claire's life even though she did not live with the children's father, presumably because she continued to care for her children and support their interaction with him.

In addition, the importance of gender for the public response to pandemic influenza was not restricted to women. Our research indicated that male gender identity was implicated in the action on influenza, as is found in other areas of health (Connell 2012). This effect was reflected in discourse on man flu, which, according to our respondents, had multiple meanings. For example, Marie commented that her father resisted illness as much as possible:

> He's the kind of man flu, right . . . You know, he won't take anything, anything at all, even the herbal stuff. He won't take anything unless he is actually in bed and crawling on the floor. And he'd have to lose his feeling to both his legs before he admitted to actually being sick at all. (Sydney, 20s, No disclosed health problems)

In this construction of man flu, Marie's father is depicted as stoic to an absurd degree, marking an investment in a hypermasculine response to nearly all infections. In their focus group research in Scotland, Hilton and Smith (2010) found that their respondents used man flu to denote severe illness, implying that an infection that affects a man must be highly virulent. We have already introduced Honigsbaum's research (2013) on newspapers and correspondence during the 1918–1919 pandemic at the end of World War I and the way in which upper-class British officers were expected to set the example of stoicism for those in the lower, less well-educated classes of soldiers. Marie's father can be said to exhibit this soldier-like resistance to infection.

In contrast, however, Lizzy seemed to imply that man flu was a source of fun:

> INTERVIEWER: A lot of people say that they've had the flu and it's just the cold.
> LIZZY: No, I have had the flu before and it's, it's, it's like the man flu! (both laugh) No it's like feelings of hot and cold and sweating and skin, your skin is sore to touch, and the other kind of symptoms . . . there's kind of no energy and really feeling all over low. (Glasgow, 20s, No disclosed health problems)

Lizzy appeared to make a joke where she teased the interviewer that her experience of influenza was man flu, but then went on to describe the severe symptoms of influenza. Vincent also made reference to man flu in a way that sponsored laughter and that seemed to point to the indeterminate experience of influenza symptoms:

INTERVIEWER: So, in terms of influenza, have you had a recent experience of influenza where you've been sick with the flu?
VINCENT: It's always a little difficult to tell when you're moving from sort of a cold [Yeah] through the man flu (Laughter) to proper influenza. [Yeah] So certainly, certainly two years ago I definitely had influenza. (Sydney, 40s, No disclosed health problems)

Vincent placed man flu between the minor effects of a cold and the severity of "proper influenza" suggesting that man flu may not be severe. Lizzy, also, appeared to set man flu apart from influenza. These uses of "man flu," then, exercised the idea that it signified the exaggeration of symptoms. Marilyn commented that man flu marked her partner's response to the common cold:

INTERVIEWER: And what about your husband? Would he go to work if he had the flu do you think?
MARILYN: No. He gets man flu, which is the common cold. [Yeah] And he does take precautions. [Yeah] But, yeah, he finds that a lot harder than me if he shuts down. [Yeah] He's got a lot of responsibilities through builders and all that kind of stuff calling on him so he would find it harder. (Melbourne, 30s, pregnant in 2009)

Marilyn's partner was represented as perhaps exaggerating the symptoms of the common cold, but also unable to absent himself from work. This version of man flu seemed to imply exaggeration mentioned by Vincent and Lizzy, but also the stoical idea of man flu to which Marie referred. Rebecca, whom we introduced in chapter 3, in speaking of her own experience with influenza symptoms, made reference to the somewhat disparaging meaning of man flu:

REBECCA: I think at the time I just kind of thought of it as just kind of a man flu thing! (laughs) You know, like, yeah, everyone gets flu, everyone has flu. I mean I've only really ever had proper flu once in my life when I really could not get out of my bed. But when you actually think of it as being that sort of illness, that level of illness, like the I.C.U. level of illness made me go, "Right that's...."

INTERVIEWER: When you say "man flu" what do you mean? (laughs)

REBECCA: Oh, you know, the overdramatizing. You've just got a bit of a cold. It's not really a big deal. Yeah, a wee day sitting on the couch sipping a Lemsip would be nice, but it's probably all it needs. It's the overdramatizing of it where you're not really that ill. (laughs) You just like to make a lot of noise about it! (laughs) (Glasgow, 30s, pregnant in 2009)

Rebecca, as did Lizzy, Vincent, and Marilyn, used "man flu" to signify the exaggeration of symptoms and implied, through the use of "man," that it denoted a male tendency to overinflate the symptoms of respiratory illness. This version of man flu also connects with our previous observations about the feminization of healthcare in connection with influenza, as men with man flu may expect that women in their lives will look after them. These divergent stoical, humorous, and exaggerating uses of "man flu" nevertheless all point to masculinity and its resonance for pandemic influenza and indeed for the social response to microbial threat in general. The ways in which "man flu" can signify a truly serious infection or be used to negotiate for care from women shows that gendered ideas of conduct are seen to be important to the self-management of pandemic influenza.

"It's all about the Baby"

Perhaps the most obvious way in which one's life trajectory intersected with the historical fact of the pandemic was the situation for pregnant women. As noted previously, it is known that pregnant women face adverse health effects in the event of a serious respiratory infection (CDC 2009). During the 2009 pandemic, however, it was observed that pregnant women made up a higher than expected proportion of admissions to intensive care units (The ANZIC Influenza Investigators 2009), alerting public health authorities that the 2009 pandemic was a particular risk for pregnant women, especially for those in the later stages of their pregnancy.

As we have discussed already in previous chapters, the pregnant women in our research had become keenly aware of this situation. Claire, Sarah, Gill, and Rebecca, among the other pregnant women we interviewed, provided accounts of how they had come to take on their "at risk" identities in the context of the 2009 pandemic. Claire noted that news media had influenced her awareness of risk: "I don't think I really appreciated what it meant for me as a pregnant woman until I saw someone do a debate on telly about whether pregnant women should be vaccinated or not" (Glasgow, 30s, Pregnant in 2009). She also mentioned an encounter with a medical practitioner and spoke of the way in which vulnerability was combined with the normative expectation of good motherhood: "The GP said, 'People like me are vulnerable, [which I'm not compared to a lot of people] and it was my responsibility to protect my unborn child from swine flu.'" As we discussed, women were aware of the duality implied in "Be alert, not alarmed" and related expectations for those in vulnerable groups, as indicated by Sarah: "'It's the flu, we'll be fine.' On the other hand, you're hearing it's a pandemic and you're pregnant and you're in an at risk group and you're going to get immunized" (Glasgow, 30s, Pregnant in 2009). There was also a sense, however, that vulnerability for pregnant women depended on the course of their pregnancy and the advent of the 2009 pandemic. Gill, for example, took precautions but was also aware that the pandemic alert lagged behind her own pregnancy: "I think by the time the recommendations came out I had given birth and it didn't bother me" (Melbourne, 30s, Pregnant in 2009). Gill's experience underlined the significance of time to those said to be vulnerable and in particular the specific way in which the advent of the pandemic in 2009 intersected with individual life trajectories.

As we noted in chapter 3 in connection with the decision to vaccinate, Rebecca said: "When you're pregnant it just becomes, everything just becomes about the baby." Rebecca also commented in her interview on the ways in which the pandemic came into her life, transforming motherhood for her and affecting the lives of her baby and children:

> suddenly you go from being the healthy, normal ones that none of this affects to being, they're now saying anyone who is pregnant or anyone who is under five should be vaccinated because they're the ones that are in danger. So yeah it is a bit scary. Again, for my children, for my baby and for my son, it was more for them it was much more, "They're the ones, they're at risk now." It is a bit of a funny thing, I mean, I've always been totally healthy. I've never had any health problems. And even being healthy, it's funny, because you get treated differently when you're pregnant but you're not unwell. There's nothing wrong with you but suddenly you're being classified as somebody who is needing to be taken care of.

[later]

It was older people, younger people and pregnancy, and babies and wee ones who were the risks. It's the first time I felt that, like, you're at risk from something, you know. It's quite a bizarre feeling, actually. It's not me being at risk again though, it's the baby being at risk. (Glasgow, 30s, Pregnant in 2009)

Rebecca provided a picture of the pandemic as a rupture in personal, family, and motherhood time. She depicted herself as experiencing at least two shifts into "at risk" status: as shifting from healthy normalcy into the surveillance applied to pregnant women per se and then, in the event of the pandemic, of a shift again into being a member of a vulnerable group with considerations for her unborn child and other children. Rebecca's narrative positioning was also strongly imbued with a normative maternal responsibility for her children, implying that her own health was only important in so far as it sustained that of her children.

Medicalized Lives

Preexisting illness was another feature of biography that was inflected with new meanings in time of pandemic. As noted, along with pregnant women, we recruited people with preexisting lung disease and with immune-related illness—mainly HIV infection—to gain insight into how vulnerable groups in the general population had engaged with the pandemic. People with chronic illness in our research had highly medicalized lives reflected in their regular engagements with clinical services and their healthcare. These connections meant that, unlike the healthy and even to some extent pregnant women, those with preexisting conditions were attached to the public health system and were directly addressed by it during the pandemic to moderate health risks. In this sense, their status as biological citizens (Petersen et al. 2010) was established for them in terms of self-identification and the everyday practicalities of managing serious chronic illness.

Those with HIV differed from those with lung disease, however. For people with HIV, the pandemic did not displace their preexisting condition; HIV remained superordinate, as Heather noted at the beginning of this chapter. If it was experienced at all, the influenza pandemic served as a way of accentuating the challenges the respondents faced in relation to HIV. For example, in this extract from a focus group with African women living in Scotland with

HIV infection, which included Heather, influenza was relegated to a lesser problem than the medical and social aspects of HIV:

HEATHER: So I think swine flu where I'm sitting doesn't really scare me, honestly, doesn't scare me at all. I'll take the necessary interventions to maybe minimize the impact it will do but it doesn't scare me. I've seen worse. I've seen so much death in my life that swine flu is another thing that is coming my way and we can deal with it. That's my attitude anyway, that's me.

INTERVIEWER: Anyone else want to say anything?

BETH: More to what Heather has said ... African people have got this hard heart, that some of the stuff people say that we are serious sometimes we don't see so maybe we have told you that we lived in ... some environments which we had to go through very hard stuff. For example, when people came, years in asylum we waited through very hard stuff, which other people cannot understand ... what we can say about all of these diseases, if you have gone through a very serious thing like hepatitis and HIV where you know that, "This is death, that's me gone" ... it's [influenza] not a thing whereby you can panic because you've gone through something very serious where you escaped death by just a corner and flu will be nothing really ...

BETH: ... compared to this thing we are in ... we could talk more about HIV ....

HEATHER: ... yes I think in essence what we are trying to say is if we had not come to the UK all of us here would be statistics ... we could all be dead if we had not found ourselves as asylum seekers in this country and where we could access medication, so what is flu? When actually I escaped death by ... by a crack or something. (Glasgow Focus Group, 30s to 50s, HIV positive)

These comments placed pandemic influenza in the context of HIV and for these women asylum seekers in their experience of dramatic uncertainty with regard to their lives. Their comments offered the view that health for them was hard won and that their focus was on survival with HIV infection. Other people with HIV infection in our research made similar comments. Matrix, noted in chapter 6, in his interview reflected on the pandemic in light of his HIV infection:

Well I suppose the HIV thing maybe (sighs) it sort of set the marker for the rest in a way it's like you know, "Once you get HIV then ... what else can you possibly get?" in terms of viral infections anyway. I mean, you might get cancer and stuff... so once that happens then other things seem to be in the background a bit. Put into the context of HIV because the HIV had such an impact sort of socially and internationally and so on... and the fear and anxiety.... I don't think these other epidemics of viruses and so on have really matched that. (Glasgow, 50s, HIV positive)

Matrix referred to HIV as providing a historical context for his engagement with pandemic influenza and perhaps in a more general sense for wider public engagements with the risks entailed. Similar dynamics of risk relativism have emerged in interviews with young injecting drug users regarding hepatitis C who spoke of HIV as a greater risk for them (Davis, Rhodes, and Martin 2004) and in the narrative of people with HIV and tuberculosis, where HIV attracted the greater stigma and tuberculosis provided a mask for HIV serostatus (Daftary 2012, Gebrekristos et al. 2009). This HIV relativism was an important frame, therefore, for the pandemic influenza engagements of people with HIV in our research and perhaps also more generally as a frame for public engagements with pandemics.

People in our research with lung disease were similarly focused on their preexisting diagnosis, but their engagement with influenza was different again because of its more direct implications. As we noted at the beginning of the chapter, Marlene who was living with lung disease commented on the news media hype and the "be alert, not alarmed" pandemic message as both, in different ways, underestimating the situation for people in her situation: "I remember being a bit upset about it 'cause I thought like I really want people to take it seriously" (Sydney, 30s, Lung disease). The critical stance of Marlene was partly attributable to the implications of a severe pandemic influenza for those with respiratory illness and the medicalized ways in which they were called on to live their lives. For example, we conducted a focus group in Melbourne with carers and people from a breathing support group who had severe, incapacitating lung disease. Some of the participants were permanently on oxygen and relied on mobility scooters, and none were able to work. One participant, Arthur, who was in his 60s and lived with his carer wife, provided a picture of the life world within which the advent of the pandemic took its meaning and effects:

My diagnosis is severe emphysema. I'm managing quite well. I have a very good carer and I have a good relationship with I think a very good GP. I have a flu vac every year. I've had Pneumovax [vaccine for infections that cause pneumonia] in the past, but I don't need it anymore because I've got future cover with the Pneumovax I understand. My complaint makes me subject to chest infections, but I have very good management of them through my GP. I send off a sputum sample and I'm very impressed with the workings of the pathology people. My GP showed me a pathology report of a sputum sample and this report gave the name of the bug that was there and also a list of five antibiotics that he could prescribe to cover that bug. So any infection I've had the medication has coped with it. So I look forward to the future with confidence because of the benefit I've had with, in the past, with medication. The treatment I've received from paramedics has been outstanding. Likewise hospital. Our Local Emergency Hospital fills all of my needs. I was most impressed with my last visit to the Local Emergency Hospital where they turned me around in only two days. In the past, we've been used to expecting to have a week in hospital with a chest infection. But the Local Emergency Hospital, Local Emergency Department are doing a great job. So I feel quite confident about what's in place healthwise. (Melbourne Focus Group, 60s to 70s, Lung disease)

People with severe lung disease, then, found pandemic influenza to be one health threat among many. As Joy, a carer from Arthur's focus group commented, for some people, their symptoms were so serious and constant that infection with pandemic influenza may have been masked. These medicalized existences are not equivalent to the experiences of others in our research, such as people with HIV who were focused on their HIV treatments and survival, or pregnant women who were engaged with norms surrounding motherhood and vaccination decisions. The deeply inscribed and variant intersectionalities of medicalized lives are illuminated in the narrative-oriented analysis we have offered here, indicating in another way how the turn to narrative in public health can be exercised in ways that reveal the complexities of living through a pandemic alert.

(In)visibilities

Another important theme of the stories our research participants related to us concerned the invisibility of vulnerability. People who may have been at greater risk of negative health outcomes if they had become infected needed to, on occasion, disclose their illness in order to explain their symptoms and or to establish hygiene and social distancing to protect themselves. This hidden dimension to vulnerability intersects with the dynamics of stigma linked with health conditions (Davis and Manderson 2014). Pandemic influenza is not popularly understood as a disease of stigmatized groups, most likely because it is an acute infection that is not bounded by group identity, though research has reported that Hispanic and Mexican people living in the United States experienced prejudice directed toward them during the 2009 event (McCauley, Minsky, and Viswanath 2013). In addition, researchers have argued that, during the pandemic, some populations ranked H1N1 as a greater stigma than HIV (Earnshaw and Quinn 2013). Telling others about vulnerability is also part of the process of taking on "at risk" identity (Davis and Manderson 2014), which flows from the discourse of pandemic preparedness and response, as we have noted previously. It is also, by implication, a process that asks the disclosee to consider themselves as "a risk" for the vulnerable. People with vulnerabilities who assert their identities and ask others in their social worlds to take action could be construed to perform biological citizenship (Petryna 2003, Rose 2007) or pandemic citizenship to establish identities, intersubjective relations, and collective responses to the threat entailed by pandemic influenza. Some of our respondents, however, found themselves called into question by those around them if they did disclose their health status. Making one's vulnerability visible was not always easy and without consequence, another way in which the public response to pandemic influenza is imbued with relations of nonequivalence.

Pregnant women in our research did not express concern with regard to their visibility and presented themselves as more exercised by their double responsibilities as expectant mothers with a duty to their own health and that of their unborn children, as we have noted. Older people, too, appeared to take on their vulnerability as part and parcel of aging and their more general focus on healthcare. Notably, the disclosure of H1N1 infection emerged as an issue in a focus group with gay men with HIV. For them, as noted, pandemic influenza was significant for the ways in which it foregrounded aspects of their HIV treatment. Nevertheless, a particularly embarrassing public disclosure appeared to have been upsetting for one man in this Glasgow focus group:

INTERVIEWER: Simon, when we sat down here you said, "Oh there's loads of similarities between HIV and swine flu" [Dean: What are they?] So what were you thinking about?

SIMON: When I got swine flu I was burnt out in my job and I got diagnosed but I couldn't get treated for it because I was too ill. But when I went to get the medication for it from the chemist, this woman was shouting my business across the shop floor and I felt like a leper just as when I was diagnosed with HIV. She said I had to have a buddy so therefore before you get swine flu you have to have a buddy?

DEAN: Before you get Tamiflu?

SIMON: Yeah. And I came here [a community group] and Karen, she went and got me the medication, otherwise I wouldn't have got it.

INTERVIEWER: Yeah

SIMON: I did complain about her conduct to the chemist which got acknowledged and then just got lost in a maze. But the similarities are pretty unreal to what I found with HIV where people just didn't want to know, you know so I just stayed indoors. It was easier than going and dealing with people. And then when I was well enough I got vaccinated for it. I didn't sort of tolerate the vaccine as good as some, if anything (laughs) it made me a lot more ill than I was before. But I just found the parallels unreal. You know you felt like shit and you needed help and no one would give you help, so. All good fun. (laughs) (Glasgow Focus Group, 30s to 50s, HIV positive)

Simon appeared to have had a negative experience in his efforts to obtain treatment and assistance for infection with H1N1. He claimed that he had been diagnosed, but it is possible that this was not done with a laboratory test and therefore was surmised on the basis of symptoms. Simon's story indicated, too, that without a buddy, he was not able to secure treatment and for this reason it was withheld until he was able to get help from his HIV support group. This account does suggest that people with significant health problems and who lack the required social capital to obtain antiviral treatment are made more vulnerable. This reinscription of vulnerability is ironic, since Simon may have been regularly taking antiviral treatment for HIV.

It also appeared to be the case that making oneself visible as vulnerable for pandemic influenza was a concern for those younger people who had chronic lung disease. People in this situation spoke of their social life as imbued with questions and experiences of disclosure and keen awareness that the healthy majority presented a risk to them of influenza transmission. In this example, Marlene commented that as someone with lung disease she was invisible to those around her:

MARLENE: Yeah, there's people who are otherwise healthy-looking adults a lot of the time so they're not an easy-to-identify group of society. Like you can see an old person, you see a pregnant person. But you can't often tell that someone has a lung disease or any other vulnerability. So yeah, I guess maybe if they had have interviewed a few people on the news like who had . . . then again, that's the media you know.

INTERVIEWER: Do you think people would take your concerns less seriously because you might appear healthy?

MARLENE: No. I don't think people take it seriously because I do appear healthy and you're exactly right: people don't understand that, yes, I might look healthy but I'm not, and I could be really unhealthy if I got this flu. It's quite difficult to get people to understand . . . yeah. It's really hard to explain to people that just because I look healthy doesn't mean I am. Especially when I put so much hard work into my health. You try to be healthy and I think and this level of health that I have is a normal person's level of health.

Marlene depicted her invisibility as a problem because those around her failed to appreciate her situation. This challenge was sharp for Marlene since she had worked hard to achieve what she termed "normal" health and therefore appeared to others to not be vulnerable in a specific way. Marlene also noted that the media had failed to make this point since it had not communicated the stories of people in her situation, a point of view that does appear to have some validity. Hilton and Hunt (2011) noted that news media during the 2009 pandemic in the United Kingdom, at least, had been relatively devoid of first-person accounts, restricted as the news was to facts and figures and the expert voice of public health authority. As we have suggested, this book helps to address this absence of personal experience narratives on pandemic influenza.

Disclosure was associated also with collective action on risk and the protection of the "at risk" by those who might pose "a risk." Cindy, a woman with lung disease who was introduced in chapter 4, reflected in her interview on disclosure and interpersonal relations in the workplace:

I've got a rather good workplace culture in terms of I've got a small department and they all know I've got lung disease. So they know that if they've got bugs, if they've got a cold . . . . Most people come to work with a cold, not the flu, but if they're capable of working, most people come. . . . They'll say, "Don't shake my hand today Cindy," or, you know, "You sit on the other side of the table during lunch." So it's good that my colleagues are aware of it and just the general mentality of the office. I'm not sure if I introduced this or it was already there and it probably just got exacerbated with me around, but we've got flexible working hours whereby working at home isn't overly encouraged but if you're feeling well enough to work but not well enough to be in the office, it's okay to work from home for that day. But more so, if you let everybody know you're contagious, so you'd prefer to work from home, everybody pretty much responds with, "Go ahead! Do everything you need to but work in the office, 'cause we don't wanna get it," you know. And I've heard that, even before I disclosed my illness to my colleagues, that mentality was there that if you're sick, don't come to work 'cause nobody else wants to get sick. (Sydney, 20s, Lung disease)

The workplace figured in pandemic influenza because it was one of the main social environments of everyday life in which infection was possible. As we considered in chapter 4, the workplace was also implied in the social distancing strategies of pandemic preparedness and response. Cindy's account referred to these concerns, but it revealed that she had been at least partly active in shaping a workplace culture where social distancing and hygiene were more likely to be enacted. Notably, this supportive culture was important to Cindy because of her health status. Disclosure—making oneself visible to others as vulnerable—was an important step in influencing relations with others.

In another context we have reflected on the emphasis on vulnerability in the discourse of pandemic preparedness and the unintended effect of splitting the healthy from the less so (Stephenson et al. 2014). This separation is significant for the public response to pandemic influenza because, as Marlene and Cindy indicated in their accounts, support from others in settings such as the workplace is vital for the health of the more vulnerable. Cindy also expressed some frustration in her interview at those people in her social experience who failed to understand her situation and, in particular, that they may present a risk to her:

INTERVIEWER: Do you think you're always constantly aware of any emerging threats out there?
CINDY: Not on a wide scale but in my daily life I certainly am. I make it an issue. 'Cause I do have a chronic cough and I make an issue that when

I deal with somebody from the public and I have a coughing fit, I just let them know, "Oh don't worry; it's not contagious—it's chronic." And I know when I sit on public transport, I hear that hacking cough at the back of the room or, you know, I deal with somebody who's sneezing, I think, "I wish they weren't at work today," or, "I wish they didn't you know, I wish there was that, that overall culture not to spread your germs." And I guess I see that because when I cough, people give me a dirty look or especially if I'm on public transport and I have a bad coughing fit, you get a few looks. And I make an effort to say, "Don't worry: it's not contagious." But for most people out there who are coughing it is contagious and I wish they weren't out in public.

Disclosure and cooperation, then, was necessary if those with specific vulnerabilities were to assert their own health needs. Such visibility, however, was not without its risks. For example, Mitzi, whom we discussed in the previous chapter, said that she was reluctant to be seen by others as "pedantic" or a "germ-freak" and spoke of admonishing her mother for being too hygienic:

They were sort of like, "Well, you know, don't go anywhere and, you know, don't . . . ." My mum's like, you know, she'll take like those Dettol wipes. You know, when you touch a shopping trolley like wipe the shopping trolley and, you know . . . . And I said, "I don't wanna be too pedantic," you know. It looks like a, you know, germ freak. (Sydney, 30s, Lung disease)

In another example of self-problematization, Pippa, introduced earlier, asked whether the interviewer thought she appeared to be a "fruit loop":

When the swine flu vaccine was coming through I rang up my GP, and like I knew that it was coming in a month, "Can I go on the waiting list to have it?" And they were going, "We're not actually having people ring up asking for waiting list status." But it's like, "Well can I make an appointment so I can be there for when it comes through." I sound like a fruit loop don't I?

It is important to recognize, then, that one of the challenges for those seeking to take precautions for influenza risk was the added burden of appearing to act outside the norm, of betraying health status or a nonnormative preoccupation with infection control. "Pedantic," "germ-freak," and "fruit-loop" mark out a public, relational dimension of efforts to respond to pandemic influenza and the implied risks of making oneself visibly concerned with infection. The disclosures we have discussed are spoken of as presenting the self as not overwhelmed by the threat of pandemic influenza, but assiduously managing health nevertheless.

The pandemic experience narratives generated in our interviews and focus groups exposed the intersectional and intersubjective qualities of real-life experiences concerning a short-lived public health emergency. The advent of the 2009 pandemic came into the life worlds of individuals, disrupting for some their biographies, while others seemed to have been scarcely troubled. Their pandemic stories engaged the temporal ordering of pandemic and personal biography, nuanced with conditions of possibility concerning age, generation, gender, preexisting illness, and intersubjective life, all of which mediated how individuals responded to microbial threat. Importantly, communications on pandemic risk that signify vulnerability mobilized also counter narrative on invulnerability, an effect that may erode efforts to address publics. The narratives show, too, the nuanced coming into being and revisable qualities of subjective life in time of pandemic. These insights attest to the benefits of the narrative approach to research on the experience of pandemics and other contagious diseases, particularly in a field where so little of such insight is available (Lin et al. 2014). In the next two chapters we consider what our narrative analysis brings to people's reflections on the pandemic and, in particular, their reading of news media hype in light of knowledge of the eventual mildness of the pandemic for most people.

References

ABC News NSW. 2009. "Swine flu warning for pregnant women: Six pregnant women in Sydney have recently been put on life support with swine flu, with health officials urging expectant mothers to take extra care [online]." ABC News NSW (ABC1 Sydney); Time: 19:05; Broadcast Date: Thursday, July 16, 2009; Duration: 1 min., 49 sec. Accessed April 5, 2017. http://search.informit.com.au.ezproxy.lib.monash.edu.au/documentSummary;dn=TEN20092800203;res=TVNEWS.

Australian Department of Health and Ageing. 2008. *Australian health management plan for pandemic influenza: Important information for all Australians*. Canberra: Australian Government, Department of Health and Ageing.

Australian Government Department of Health and Ageing. 2011. *Review of Australia's health sector response to pandemic (H1N1) 2009: Lessons identified*. Canberra: Commonwealth of Australia.

CDC. 2009. "Novel Influenza A (H1N1) virus infections in three pregnant women—United States, April–May 2009." *MMWR Dispatch*. Atlanta.

Connell, R. 2012. "Gender, health and theory: Conceptualizing the issue, in local and world perspective." *Social Science & Medicine* 74 (11):1675–1683.
Conrad, P. 2013. "Medicalization: Changing contours, characteristics, and contexts." In *Medical sociology on the move*, edited by W Cockerham, 195–214. Dordrecht: Springer.
Daftary, A. 2012. "HIV and tuberculosis: The construction and management of double stigma." *Social Science & Medicine* 74 (10):1512–1519.
Davies, B, and R Harre. 1990. "Positioning: The discursive production of selves." *Journal for the Theory of Social Behaviour* 20 (1):43–63.
Davis, M, and L Manderson, eds. 2014. *Disclosure in health and illness*. Abingdon: Routledge.
Davis, M, T Rhodes, and A Martin. 2004. "Preventing hepatitis C: 'Common sense,' 'the bug' and other perspectives from the risk narratives of people who inject drugs." *Social Science and Medicine* 59:1807–1818.
Department of Health United Kingdom. 2007. *Pandemic flu: A national framework for responding to an influenza pandemic*. London: Author.
Earnshaw, V, and D Quinn. 2013. "Influenza stigma during the 2009 H1N1 pandemic." *Journal of Applied Social Psychology* 43 (S1):E109–E114. doi: 10.1111/jasp.12049.
Frank, A. 1995. *The wounded storyteller: Body, illness and ethics*. Chicago: University of Chicago Press.
Gebrekristos, H, M Lurie, N Mthethwa, and Q Karim. 2009. "Disclosure of HIV status: Experiences of patients enrolled in an integrated TB and HAART pilot programme in South Africa." *African Journal of AIDS Research* 8 (1):1–6.
Hankivsky, O. 2012. "Women's health, men's health, and gender and health: Implications of intersectionality." *Social Science & Medicine* 74 (11):1712–1720.
Hilton, S, and K Hunt. 2011. "UK newspapers' representation of the 2009–10 outbreak of swine flu: One health scare not over-hyped by the media?" *Journal of Epidemiology and Community Health* 65:941–946.
Hilton, S, and E Smith. 2010. "Public views of the UK media and government reaction to the 2009 swine flu pandemic." *BMC Public Health* 10:697.
Hine, D. 2010. *The 2009 influenza pandemic: An independent review of the UK response to the 2009 influenza pandemic*. London: Pandemic Flu Response Review Team, Cabinet Office.
Honigsbaum, M. 2013. "Regulating the 1918–19 pandemic: Flu, stoicism and the Northcliffe Press." *Medical History* 57 (2):165–185. doi: http:/dx.doi.org/10.1017/mdh.2012.101.
Hyden, L, and J Brockmeier. 2008. "Introduction: From the retold to the performed story." In *Health, illness and culture: Broken narratives*, edited by L Hyden and J Brockmeier, 1–15. New York: Routledge.
Kilbourne, E. 2006. "Influenza pandemics of the 20th century." *Emerging Infectious Diseases* 12 (1):9–14.
Lin, L, E Savoia, F Agboola, and K Viswanath. 2014. "What have we learned about communication inequalities during the H1N1 pandemic: A systematic review of the literature." *BMC Public Health* 14 (1):484. doi: 10.1186/1471-2458-14-484.
McCauley, M, S Minsky, and K Viswanath. 2013. "The H1N1 pandemic: Media frames, stigmatization and coping." *BMC Public Health* 13 (1):1116. doi: http://dx.doi.org/10.1186/1471-2458-13-1116.
Petersen, A, M Davis, S Fraser, and J Lindsay. 2010. "Healthy living and citizenship: An overview." *Critical Public Health* 20 (4):391–400.

Petryna, A 2003. *Life exposed: Biological citizens after Chernobyl*. Princeton: Princeton University Press.
Rose, N. 2007. *The politics of life itself: Biomedicine, power and subjectivity in the twenty-first century*. Princeton: Princeton University Press.
Stephenson, N, M Davis, P Flowers, E Waller, and C MacGregor. 2014. "Mobilising 'vulnerability' in the public health response to pandemic influenza." *Social Science & Medicine* 102:10–17.
The ANZIC Influenza Investigators. 2009. "Critical Care Services and 2009 H1N1 Influenza in Australia and New Zealand." *New England Journal of Medicine* 361 (20):1925–1934. doi: 10.1056/NEJMoa0908481.

7
News Media Hype?

> I don't think I ever thought about, "Oh my God I might get that."
> I think that I'm so used to thinking about how it would affect other
> people and I don't think I really appreciated about what it meant
> for me as a pregnant woman until I saw someone do a debate on
> telly about whether pregnant women should be vaccinated or not.
> (Claire, Glasgow, 30s, Pregnant in 2009)

Research has indicated that news media were pivotal to awareness of the 2009 influenza pandemic (Lin et al. 2014), even among those with severe respiratory illness and therefore connected with the health system (Hutchinson et al. 2010). In what follows we explore our participants' accounts of news media messages and, if need be, how they put advice into action. We develop an account of what we call "persuasion narrative" that was sustained in this storytelling, with its dominant features of self-address, self-questioning, and gradual self-recognition, as demonstrated in Claire's comments beginning this chapter and echoed in Sarah's exclamation, "That could be me!" discussed in chapter 2. This elaboration of persuasion narrative is an important step in our argument given the narrative turn in public health.

This chapter also picks up a point we made in chapter 2 regarding the narrative nexus (Mairal 2011), formed by news, pandemics, and the public interest, and the related notion that stories of an emerging and threatening pandemic are archly newsworthy. News media on the 2009 pandemic was prominent in the accounts of our research participants and was one reason for the development of our argument on the significance of narrative to public engagements with pandemic threat. Analysis of pandemic narratives, therefore, would be incomplete without due consideration of the role of news media.

It was the case, too, that news on the 2009 pandemic was an important feature of the social response across nations and the world and was central to public health efforts. As we have indicated in previous chapters, advertising,

Pandemics, Publics, and Narrative. Mark Davis and Davina Lohm, Oxford University Press (2020).
© Oxford University Press.
DOI: 10.1093/oso/9780190683764.001.0001

electronic and printed information, telephone triage, and press releases and conferences were used to create awareness of the pandemic and to advise publics on how to act on health risks. Public health used these strategies to avoid or moderate counterproductive responses, such as resistance to vaccines or negative reactions to the manner in which public health systems conduct themselves. Communications strategies also feature in public health's address to itself and, in particular, the knowledge systems that sustain it as a social institution. Likewise, our interviewees referred to news media alongside other forms of information and advice emanating from expert sources. As we will see, too, quotations and videos of experts providing facts and information were a prominent feature of the news itself.

Social research on health media is commonly framed by the notion of message coding, transmission, and reception and conceptualizations of how message content can influence individual risk perception, motivation, and behavior (MacDonald et al. 2013). Departing from the mediation framing of health communications, we assume that media are entangled with lived experience and action on health (Kember and Zylinska 2015), and that media make public health narratives available to publics for their own consumption and recirculation. Drawing on concepts from biological citizenship (Petryna 2003, Rose 2007), and biocommunicability (Briggs and Nichter 2009), we focus attention on the particular ways in which the public health messages on pandemic influenza became part of the social worlds of members of the general public and, therefore, how their experiences took form. We attend to the institutional interests of public health, the technologies and practices of media, and the material, biographical and cultural circumstances in which publics decode, transform, or ignore messages.

It is often argued that news media exaggerate risks or distort information in ways that may mislead audiences, though these perspectives tend to assume that expert knowledge is stable and uncontestable and that audiences are easily manipulable (Kitzinger 1999). Some have argued that news media and popular culture more generally are not likely to always serve public health because ideology and economic factors also shape how news, for example, is produced and circulated (Kline 2006). Moreover, news media have been shown to sustain a gendered bias in expert authority by featuring mainly male experts (Niemi and Pitkanen 2017), underlining how news reporting can reinforce social norms over and above the actual content of news items. As we will see, news texts on the 2009 pandemic in the United Kingdom and Australia were factual and featured the voices of experts, and therefore appeared to evade some aspects of the risk exaggeration critique. Paradoxically, however, our research participants, consistent with the findings of others in the field (Hilton and Smith 2010, Holland and Blood 2012), spoke of news media hype when recalling the news in 2009. In what follows we aim to reconcile this apparent contradiction with reference to concepts from narrative theory.

This chapter begins with an overview of the news media response to the 2009 pandemic event in the United Kingdom and Australia, which, as will become clear, was remarkable in its own right. We explore research on news media that reveals these texts to have relied mostly on the authoritative commentary provided by experts in the field, in contrast with perspectives from our research participants where they argued that media hyped news on the pandemic. We conclude with some reflections on how, in light of this apparent media hype, our informants created narrative on how they were persuaded into acceptance of being "at risk," where relevant. This chapter, therefore, addresses the concept of narrative persuasion by considering how our research participants addressed themselves to the narrative and news media complexities of the pandemic situation in 2009.

News Media Stories on Pandemic wwInfluenza

Reflecting the news worthiness of the 2009 pandemic, news media activity during the pandemic was extraordinarily large, easily outstripping activity for other health problems. Data and several examples help to illustrate the scale and tenor of the news media on the early pandemic. *Newsbank* collates news items from printed and online newspapers, blogs, newswires, journals, broadcast transcripts, and videos from just under 10,000 sources around the globe, as of April 2017 (6,692 from North America). Table 7.1 shows that in

Table 7.1 Frequency of News Stories over Time—World (8,000+ Sources)

	2008	2009	2014
"swine flu"	158	198,649	5,156
"breast cancer"	106,262	124,617	107,756
"HIV"	64,568	73,520	75,502
"superbugs"	1,851	1,317	1,871

Table 7.2 Frequency of News Stories over Time—Australia (448 Sources)

	2008	2009	2014
"swine flu"	1	10,344	162
"breast cancer"	6,901	7,771	8,248
"HIV"	1,804	1,728	1,748
"superbugs"	82	95	134

2008, there were 158 news items worldwide that used the term "swine flu." In 2009, however, there were 198,649 items, and by 2014, the annual frequency had dropped to 5,156 items. Table 7.1 also shows that in comparison to frequency counts for "breast cancer," "HIV," and "superbugs," the swine flu news story in 2009 was distinctive for being sudden and large, but short-lived. The patterns for news media in the United Kingdom and Australia were similar (see Tables 7.2 and 7.3). The H1N1 pandemic also seems to have been a prominent news story compared with other recent microbial threats, for example, there were 15,954 news items on "bird flu" during the 2004 outbreak of H1N5, 107,862 items on SARS in 2002–2003, and 122,310 items on Zika virus in 2016. Ebola alone eclipsed swine flu's 2009 count of 198,649 items, with 210,630 items in 2014, though the *Newsbank* data base has also grown since 2009.

Early reporting on the 2009 pandemic was distinctive for picking up on the World Health Organization (WHO) announcement on April 25, 2009, of a "public health emergency of international concern" and digesting this message for publics as a health "alert." Table 7.4 displays indicative headlines from April 26 and 27, 2009, in high-circulation newspapers from Australia and Scotland.

Table 7.3 Frequency of News Stories over Time—United Kingdom (476 Sources)

	2008	2009	2014
"swine flu"	1	24,131	460
"breast cancer"	9,240	10,178	13,475
"HIV"	5,751	6,282	7,133
"superbugs"	1,183	689	502

Table 7.4 Example Newspaper Headlines on H1N1, from Victoria, NSW and Scotland, April 26–27, 2009

Date	Headline	Newspaper	State, Country
April 26	"Swine flu kills 60"	Sunday Herald	Victoria, Australia
April 27	"Doctors sound alarm on pig flu"	The Age	Victoria, Australia
April 26	"Pandemic alert: 60 dead, 1000 ill"	Sunday Telegraph	NSW, Australia
April 26	"Spectre of pandemic: Nation shut down as flu kills 61"	Sun Herald	NSW, Australia
April 26	"Alert on killer flu"	Sunday Mail	Scotland
April 26	"Mexican swine flu is "potential pandemic" WHO considers declaring international emergency"	Herald and the Sunday Herald	Scotland

Source: Newsbank.

These stories were among the first news items on the pandemic, and they captured the moment when the WHO announced the public health emergency. These news items contained a smattering of words that connoted threat, such as "deadly" and "red alert," but they were dominated by quotations from public health authorities, including the director general of the WHO. They relayed facts pertaining to the outbreak in Mexico, what was done there to address the spread of infection and care for those infected, and provided some advice on what members of the general public could do to avoid infection.

News Media Frames

Framing analyses from this period show that the newspapers and television news in particular avoided sensationalism and reported the pandemic soberly and scientifically. Framing analysis involves identifying the ways in which texts use language and images to shape knowledge (Kitzinger 2007). Hilton and Hunt (2011) content analyzed 2,374 articles published in the United Kingdom between March 1, 2009, and February 28, 2010, and concluded that inflammatory discourse was avoided in favor of reporting facts prepared by health authorities and advising the general public on prevention, treatment, and vaccination. As with previous news media research on Avian influenza (Ungar 2008) and emerging infectious diseases in general (Shih, Wijaya, and Brossard 2008), Hilton and Hunt found that the narrative organization of the news on H1N1 shifted over time from an alert in the first few days to ongoing reassurance of the public. Hilton and Hunt found that early reporting on the pandemic referred to previous pandemics such as the one in 1918–1919 and that the frequency of news items mirrored the first peak of cases in the United Kingdom in July 2009, followed by declining interest over the following months, consistent with the data presented previously. They also noted the absence of personal stories of experience with the infection and the dominance of fact-based statements from public health authorities. Hilton and Hunt made the point that news media are often regarded as an undesirable source of information on health because commercial and other interests influence how stories are framed, a view that was not sustained in their own analysis. They concluded that the news media, in the case of the 2009 pandemic at least, did appear to be have been effective transmitters of facts and useful advice for publics.

A content analysis of the Australian television news stories made a similar point. Fogarty et al. (2011) found that televised news items from 2009 established a balance between expressing the potential seriousness of the pandemic without encouraging overreaction. They found that, among the reporting of facts regarding the number of people infected and the spread of the virus, were messages of the need for calm and that the government was effectively managing the situation. In a close focus content analysis of three major Australian newspapers from the period, Holland and Blood (2010) found that pandemic news stories peaked in the week of April 27, 2009, two days after the WHO's announcement of a "public health emergency of international concern." As in their related research on television news, Holland and Blood found that the print media were tempered, and typically used sources from public health professionals such as chief medical officers in Australian states. Their analysis also showed, however, that the stories were also somewhat narratively open and unresolved, conveying the message of calm and reassurance at times in tandem with messages that the pandemic could develop into something more serious. Holland and Blood showed that the early pandemic news story, at heart, was an inchoate assemblage of fact and uncertainty, a narrative terrain that public health communications helped to artfully negotiate. This narrative openness indicates, also, that the pandemic news story had an emergent, fluid quality in its early days and weeks. Publics were therefore invited to consider this temporarily open-ended story, which reverberated into future news stories and other storytelling practices, including the interviews and focus groups we conducted.

Fear Mongering?

The factual, calming content of news stories on the pandemic, however, were not the only messages publics received. Hilton and Smith (2010) made the point that, while their research of newspaper content found little evidence of fact distortion and the encouragement of panic, members of the general public did say that the media were prone to "overreport" the pandemic, much like many of our respondents. Hilton and Smith conducted focus groups in Scotland between October 2009 and January 2010, using a sampling approach similar to ours. Their respondents, like ours, confirmed that media were their main source of information on the pandemic. Hilton and Smith attribute the finding that their research participants had found the news to have overreported the pandemic to the scale of news reporting, which as we have seen, was sudden and large in comparison to other health issues. Indeed, Hilton and Smith's respondents reported feeling overwhelmed by the reporting. Like Hilton and Smith, Holland and Blood (2012) mirrored their content analyses of news media with interviews and focus groups conducted in Melbourne, Sydney, and Canberra in the period from August 2009 to September 2010. They also used a sampling approach similar to Hilton and Smith and ourselves. Consistent with the Scottish focus groups and our research, Holland and Blood's respondents expressed distrust, not of the action of governments during the pandemic, but of a "fear-mongering" media. A meta-analysis of survey results from the United Kingdom also concluded that audiences had found that the media had "made too much fuss" (Rubin et al. 2015, page 1554).

Exemplifying this notional media hype, one of the focus groups we conducted with people under 30 years of age in Melbourne (only one of whom had chronic lung disease, in this particular case a mild form), demonstrated awareness of the scale of news reporting on the pandemic but also how the pandemic narrative informed the respondents' reception of the news reporting. They also noted that, perhaps due to its lack of immediate health threat for most of them, the news stories could be "exciting" and perhaps even a form of entertainment:

INTERVIEWER: So how did you hear about the swine flu?
LACHLAN: The media whip-up on the news. News stories everywhere. Yeah, I guess it's what came across the news and the papers, and things like that.
JASON: Yeah, that's about it, yeah. News, all over the news. A hot topic for a couple of weeks.
INTERVIEWER: So what sort of things were you hearing on the news?
LACHLAN: Pandemic. How scary it was.
JASON: It's spreading. People are dying. First case in Australia. First this, first that.
LACHLAN: It sounded a bit like the movie *Outbreak*. I mean it's quite exciting to hear words like that. [Laughter] But . . . "airborne," you know. Quite exciting. It seemed like a big beat-up, but, definitely, there was a lot of presence in the media about it.
INTERVIEWER: Yep. So did you do anything in particular to find out about it? Did any of you hunt up on the Internet or speak to a doctor, or anything? [No]
LACHLAN: No, not really. I think I looked at it 'cause I knew it would come up in pub trivia on Wednesdays. [And it did] H1N1, I didn't actually know what they stood for. That's what it got called, H1N1.
INTERVIEWER: That's what it was, yep, H1N1. So you remembered it for the trivia?
LACHLAN: Yeah, that was probably the only reason. Just read it through the papers. I tend to be an addict of *The Age* anyway so I read every article that seems to pop up. (Melbourne Focus Group, 20s, No disclosed health problems)

Lachlan and his focus group colleagues did not depict themselves as personally addressed by the danger of the pandemic. The stories of the emerging pandemic had a distant quality, and the participants took the position of observers, recalling comments we made in chapter 4 on social distance from the pandemic. Notably, Lachlan connected news media on the pandemic with filmic portrayals of contagion and its social effects, underlining the point previously made that messages on a particular pandemic are read in the context of a ramifying and well-understood popular culture on pandemics (Davis 2017). It is important to recognize, then, that the actual content of a particular news story or a whole period of reporting may be fitted into a preexisting narrative context (Seale 2002, Ungar 2000) and that therefore meaning is not only found in the content of particular news texts but in the life of pandemic narrative in the social worlds of audiences.

In their couple interview, Liz and Peter, who were in their early 60s and lived on the outskirts of Melbourne, also commented that the news media had told a story of panic:

INTERVIEWER: What I want you to do now is think a little bit about 2009 and swine flu. What can you remember about it?

PETER: Publicity. A bit of panic. And going about my own business thinking it'll never affect me anyway 'cause I am not flying overseas and I'm not associating with people who I think might have it. Pretty simplistic but yeah, get on with life.

LIZ: Yeah. I remember similar too like the Asian countries seemed to be affected by it, I remember. And thinking it could be scary if you start to think that things are passed on from animals to humans and how they mutate. But I wasn't alarmed, but I can remember a lot of publicity about how dangerous it was, and how easily it was spreading.

INTERVIEWER: Can you remember anything about the type of publicity, the sorts of things that you were hearing?

LIZ: Always panic.

PETER: Always panic. Always bad news. Always more people being affected by it or a particular person who's come to Australia who's got it and they've been isolated. And there's always panic, you know, "any second now." The press were waiting I think with bated breath, hoping that a million people would drop dead so they could sell more papers. And it's just a build-up of panic. That's what I remember and thinking, "It can't be that bad. We haven't been warned to wear masks or anything else. So, you know, it's just a beat-up, basically."

INTERVIEWER: So were you concerned about it?

PETER: Not at all. Not at all.

LIZ: No. (Melbourne, 50s, No disclosed health problems)

Importantly, the so-called panicky news stories did not inspire panic in Liz and Peter. Like Lachlan and his focus group colleagues, Liz and Peter observed the story at a distance; they were aware of the events and watched the story unfold but did not expect that they would become part of it. Their imagined distance from the center of the story was underlined by Liz's comment that Asian countries were more severely affected, locating the threat beyond Australian borders and inscribing life in Melbourne as far removed and therefore safe from microbial threat. This way of signifying risk was at odds with news reports that Melbourne, for a few weeks in 2009, had the highest prevalence rate of H1N1 notifications anywhere in the world (Wilson 2009).

The public view that news media hyped the pandemic in contrast with the actual content of the news texts indicated that publics responded to media using their own framings derived from their lifetime experience of pandemic narratives and preconceptions of media as prone to hype the news. Assessments of overreporting and fear-mongering therefore reflected what audiences brought with them into their interpretation of news media stories. As news texts are potentially read in the context of previous texts (Ungar 2000), it may have also been the case that the early news stories—which as we have seen communicated WHO's announcement of public health emergency—set the narrative frame for subsequent news stories, even those which restricted themselves to factual reporting and sound advice. That is, while the reporting was sober and factual, it was read inside the pretext of a pandemic threat established in the very early days of reporting and resonating with previous pandemics and a more general, well-established narrative on pandemic threat.

In addition, media do not only influence individuals through their texts; the form and structure of address and reception—in this case the enormous number of news items and seeming ubiquity of the pandemic message—also impinge on audiences. As we have seen, the news message on the public health emergency was, for a time, itself a pandemic of a kind. Publics, therefore, may have responded to the repetition of the message across media as a message in itself of the potential severity of the pandemic and therefore found the media to be overly active.

Also, publics may have found the media to have hyped the pandemic because of the narrative structure of the news items and in particular the different "voices"—speaking positions and or characters—discernible in the narratives, including that of the narrator (Squire et al. 2014). Wagner-Egger et al.'s (2011) analysis of public perceptions of swine flu news media in Switzerland showed that medical experts were construed as heroic, while the news media was seen as the source of villainy. Hilton and Hunt (2011) and Fogarty et al. (2011) have noted that public health experts were recurrent sources of information in news stories. These figures were often quoted and therefore were seen to "speak" in these news texts and therefore appear as characters in the pandemic story. But the journalist authors of the news texts also had their own more or less hidden voices, in contrast to the apparent voices of the quoted public health experts. News texts then mobilized public health actors as heroes, but also by implication the voice and implied figure of the media itself as an agent in the pandemic narrative, reporting facts but also sustaining the possibility of a viral breakthrough, if not quite acting out the role of pandemic villain. Conceivably, publics also responded to these different characters of the pandemic news story, finding public health officials to be sober and fact-oriented, along with the hidden and not so hidden "persona" of the media as nevertheless persisting with the story of a possible catastrophe.

Persuasion Narrative

Pandemic news, then, has many elements, among them the interests of public health to provide facts and calm the population; the investments of news media in the sensational story; how a public is imagined to be interested in a pandemic; how publics are convened as subject to pandemic; how communications shape biopolitical identities and action; how publics might receive a message on a pandemic; the mixtures of fact, fiction, voice and character that help to narrativize a pandemic; and how messages come into the life worlds of audiences. Key for this analysis of pandemic news stories is their role in the establishment of novel self-engagement. As Judith Butler has put it, "it is by being interpellated within the terms of language that a certain social existence of the body first becomes possible" (Butler 1997, page 5). We have previously noted, through the examples of Cameron (chapter 1), Sarah (chapter 2), Mary (chapter 3), and others, how people in our research came to view themselves differently because of the pandemic and news about it. Cameron gave us his infection story and Sarah her epiphany of self-recognition—"That could be me!"—tied to news media messages regarding pregnant women. Mary used similar language—"That could happen to me"—in connection with her discussion of a television advertisement. In what follows we expand on these examples through further material from our research that helps to establish what we refer to as "persuasion narrative," that is, personal experience narrative on transformed self-awareness and conditional acceptance of personal pandemic threat. We adopt the term "persuasion narrative" as a deliberate and, we hope, productive reversal of the more common notion of "narrative persuasion," noted in chapter 2. The analysis we develop aims to value how narrative might persuade but also how individuals may also rework, redeploy, or resist narrative to fit their own circumstances, assumptions, and preferences. We think that critical examination of persuasion narrative fits with the aim of a more just and effective response to the microbial threats to life, helping to bring publics and public health into closer alignment and creative engagement (Wald 2008). We focus mainly on news stories in this chapter, but the analysis has salience for narrative approaches to public health in general.

Claire, noted at the beginning of this chapter, recalled her growing awareness of the pandemic in a manner that resonated with the accounts provided by Mary, Sarah, and Cameron. Like them, Claire created a narrative of self-persuasion into her position as an "at-risk" subject. Claire emphasized this positioning by at first explaining her resistance:

INTERVIEWER: So can you remember when you first heard about it? (H1N1)
CLAIRE: I can remember seeing something about China and they were walking about with masks and it was on telly and I just thought "What the hell is going on here?" and then they said that it had hit Britain and then they had these surnames of people in Britain who had had it and some had survived it and some hadn't and . . . I can remember thinking "Swine flu? How can anyone get Swine Flu, do pigs not get it?!" (laughs) But then I knew that it had been passed from pigs to humans and it had already spread more widely and I just thought, "Oh my God, if someone gets that it will be really serious" but I don't think I ever thought about, "Oh my God I might get that." I think that I'm so used to thinking about how it would affect other people and I don't think I really appreciated about what it meant for me as a pregnant woman until I saw someone do a debate on telly about whether pregnant women should be vaccinated or not. (Glasgow, 30s, Pregnant in 2009)

Claire depicted herself as someone whose awareness of being at personal risk evolved as a matter of accumulating knowledge. The televised debate was put forward as the media event that had most resonance—partly because of what had preceded it—and which led her to take on the notion that, like some pregnant women, she may have been at risk and that vaccination may be wise. Claire's account narrated a transition from a general threat to a personal, particular, one. Her account revealed some of the complexity of media environments, since she made mention of news and a current affairs debate, which, along with the other examples noted throughout this book, reinforced media multiplicity. In this way, Claire, like Cameron, Sarah, and

Mary, performed narrative interpellation; the moment of personal realization of becoming at risk of the pandemic. These accounts showed how news media and other communications on pandemic risk come into and combine in life worlds with significant effects on biopolitical identities and action on health. These accounts show how experience of the pandemic is entangled with news media, in particular.

This persuasion narrative was also identifiable in the interviews of those who had no specific risk of serious disease if infected. Vaughn, a Sydney-sider in his 20s and self-disclosed as healthy, also took the position of someone who was critical of the pandemic message. His account made connections between news of the 2009 pandemic and the Spanish Influenza pandemic:

INTERVIEWER: Do you remember anything about the media back in 2009?
VAUGHN: I remember it was in the news a lot because it was sort of an unknown. It was like, "Is this gonna be like the Spanish flu?" Or yeah, I think there's always, well for me anyway, I always have like a bit of cynicism with whatever, well skepticism is a better word for whatever the media is saying about sort of stuff to do with health especially. I think that sort of rings alarm bells when they say the world is under attack from a pandemic or terrorists are all coming to get us, or whatever it might be. So I do remember quite a bit of hype about it. It's justified to an extent, but where that line is in the sand I don't know. And again, the medical practitioners will be the ones that will be doing press releases and all that sort of stuff. It starts to get interesting when Tamiflu producers start doing press releases and that is becoming media content. But I don't know enough about it, to be honest. I don't think it's hype if people are dying. If it's evident that it exists and the science knows that it can spread really easily then that's not hype—that makes sense. But again it's where do you draw the line in the sand? I mean has it the potential to be absolutely terrible? But it's not, so yeah. (Sydney, 40s, No disclosed health problems)

Like the previously discussed participants, Vaughn used a question to emphasize his position on news of the pandemic threat, "Is this gonna be like the Spanish flu?" Vaughn's question established him as a knowing, reflexive subject, in his case, engaged with knowledge of the seriousness of the 1918–1919 pandemic and the question of the relative severity of the emerging 2009 pandemic. Vaughn's articulation of skepticism echoed an approach that recurred across interviews and focus groups in our research (Davis et al. 2014) and other research conducted in Scotland (Hilton and Smith 2010) and Australia (Holland and Blood 2012), as previously discussed. His use of the "line in the sand" metaphor signaled that Vaughn was aware that authorities faced a problem when pandemic warnings turn out to be false alarms.

Persuasion narrative also offers a way to reframe the skeptical reception of the news media stories on the pandemic, which, remarkably enough, transpired with journalists and editors only rarely having to signify hype in the textual content of news stories (Hilton and Hunt 2011, Holland et al. 2012) since the cumulative scale and temporal rhythm of these stories spoke of the pandemic. Talk of media hype can be seen as an effect of persuasion narrative in the sense that it reflects the suspended judgment of publics who adopt a "wait and see" approach. Persuasion narrative mobilizes skepticism, drawing in the commonly recognized idea that media use hype to sell their stories and also the culture of pandemic narrative that exercises fact and fiction so creatively and extensively. Persuasion narrative, however, runs deeper than simply offering a way of framing the news media as self-interested panic merchants. The accounts offered by people in our research indicate that news media help to constitute experience of the pandemic and are implicated in the transformation and establishment of biopolitical identities, such as "at risk" or "infected." Publics may therefore benefit from seeing news media as hyped, treating it with skepticism, and not rushing to judgement and action. This self-protective distancing is in part achieved through persuasion narrative, which offers narrators the position of a reflexive, astute subject but without closing off the possibility that the pandemic might in the end turn out to be "real," as it did, in different ways, for many of our respondents.

As we have argued, the ways in which our participants spoke of discovering themselves as at risk or, as in Cameron's case, presumably infected, connects with the narrative turn in health communications on matters such as pandemics, microbial threats, and vaccines. Our analysis suggests that subjects bring interpretion skills to health messages and news media, a view that is consistent with narrative theory in general (Andrews, Tamboukou, and Squire 2013). They put stories together themselves to explain their particular circumstances and to open to view the questions that pertain to the personal realities of a pandemic. They show themselves to be carefully skeptical but wisely flexible. They suggest narrative engagements with public health, which affords them some scope for astute resistance or carefully accepted at-risk identity, much in the way illness narratives are said to open up possibilities for struggles with other health conditions (Charon 2006, Frank 1995, Greenhalgh 2006, Kleinman 1988). They distinguish between what they see as expert advice and media storytelling, indicating engagements with narrative polysemia but also an overall skepticism. Recognizing oneself in this complex storytelling is not a simple matter, but one that is itself narratively organized as Sarah, Mary, Claire, Cameron, and Vaughn indicated in their questioning self-recognition as individuals affected by the pandemic in 2009. The idea that narrative can be used by the public health system to persuade, then, underestimates the panoply of pandemic storytelling that is possible and how individuals exploit narrative becoming to carefully explore the transformation of their identities. In so doing, they reserve for themselves some forms of control over an impending threat over which they may have little power, ultimately, to resist. In this view, health communications could be conceptualized as ways of expanding the interpretive options of publics, providing tools and techniques that enable them to navigate a particular pandemic or infectious diseases in general.

It does appear, though, that this account of persuasion narrative runs counter to currents in health communications, some of which trends to schematic and paternalistic delimiting of ways of thinking and acting on health problems. There is then a wider debate to be had of the publicness of public health and the claims on volition that pandemic subjects might care to exercise. This debate links to the ways in which pandemic preparedness and response is heavily inflected with securitization (Lakoff 2008, 2015), which in turn connects with the various biopolitical rationalities associated with pandemics of the twentieth and twenty-first centuries: Spanish Influenza and the stoical Edwardians on war footing (Honigsbaum 2013); polio and dutiful Cold War citizens (Martin 1994); HIV and flexible risk subjects (Lupton 1999).

Our analysis also suggests that media hype on pandemic news is the starting point for publics, despite the observation that news items for the most part are expert driven, factual, and sober. Publics appear to have a critical orientation to news that precedes and exceeds any one pandemic event. Efforts to influence publics through news media, at least, will need to take this situation into account. These challenges were all the more acute in 2009 because the pandemic turned out to be far milder than first thought, raising deep questions of uncertainty, trust, and how to best engage publics. We turn to these aspects of our analysis in next chapter.

References

Andrews, M, M Tamboukou, and C Squire, eds. 2013. *Doing narrative research, second edition*. London: Sage.

Briggs, C, and M Nichter. 2009. "Biocommunicability and the biopolitics of pandemic threats." *Medical Anthropology* 28 (3):189–198.

Butler, J. 1997. *Excitable speech: A politics of the performative*. London: Routledge.

Charon, R. 2006. *Narrative medicine: Honoring the stories of illness*. New York: Oxford University Press.

Davis, M. 2017. "'Is it going to be real?' Narrative and media on a pandemic." *Forum Qualitative Sozialforschung / Forum: Qualitative Social Research* 18 (1, http://nbn-resolving.de/urn:nbn:de:0114-fqs1701187).

Davis, M, P Flowers, D Lohm, E Waller, and N Stephenson. 2014. "'We became sceptics': Fear and media hype in general public narrative on the advent of pandemic influenza." *Sociological Inquiry* 84 (3):499–518.

Fogarty, A, K Holland, M Imison, R Blodd, S Chapman, and S Holding. 2011. "Communicating uncertainty—how Australian television reported H1N1 risk in 2009: A content analysis." *BMC Public Health* 11:181.

Frank, A. 1995. *The wounded storyteller: Body, illness and ethics*. Chicago: University of Chicago Press.

Greenhalgh, T 2006. *What seems to be the trouble? Stories in illness and healthcare*. Oxford: Radcliffe Publishing.

Hilton, S, and K Hunt. 2011. "UK newspapers" representation of the 2009–10 outbreak of swine flu: One health scare not over-hyped by the media?" *Journal of Epidemiology and Community Health* 65:941–946.

Hilton, S, and E Smith. 2010. "Public views of the UK media and government reaction to the 2009 swine flu pandemic." *BMC Public Health* 10:697.

Holland, K, and R Blood. 2010. "Not just another flu? The framing of swine flu in the Australian Press in Media, Democracy and Change: Refereed Proceedings of the Australian and New Zealand Communications Association Annual Conference, Canberra July 7–9."

Holland, K, and W Blood. 2012. "Public responses and reflexivity during the Swine flu pandemic in Australia." *Journalism Studies* 14 (4):523–538. iFirst: doi:10.1080/1461670X.2012.744552.

Holland, K, W Blood, M Imison, S Chapman, and A Fogarty. 2012. "Risk, expert uncertainty, and Australian news media: Public and private faces of expert opinion during the 2009 swine flu pandemic." *Journal of Risk Research* 15 (6):657–671. doi: 10.1080/13669877.2011.652651.

Honigsbaum, M. 2013. "Regulating the 1918–19 pandemic: Flu, stoicism and the Northcliffe Press." *Medical History* 57 (2):165–185. doi: http://dx.doi.org/10.1017/mdh.2012.101.

Hutchinson, AF, MA Thompson, L Clark, LB Irving, AF Hutchinson, MA Thompson, L Clark, and LB Irving. 2010. "Communicating information regarding human H1N1-09 virus to high-risk consumers: Knowledge and understanding of COPD patients in Melbourne, Australia." *Collegian: Journal of the Royal College of Nursing, Australia* 17 (4):199–205.

Kember, S, and J Zylinska. 2015. *Life after new media: Mediation as a vital process*. Cambridge, MA: MIT Press.

Kitzinger, J. 1999. "Researching risk and the media." *Health, Risk & Society* 1 (1):55–69.
Kitzinger, J. 2007. "Framing and frame analysis." In *Media studies: Key issues and debates*, edited by E Devereux, 129–150. London: Sage.
Kleinman, A. 1988. *The illness narratives: Suffering, healing and the human condition*. New York: Basic Books.
Kline, K. 2006. "A decade of research on health content in the media: The focus on health challenges and sociocultural context and attendant informational and ideological problems." *Journal of Health Communication* 11 (1):43–59.
Lakoff, A. 2008. "The generic biothreat, or, how we became unprepared." *Cultural Anthropology* 23 (3):399–428.
Lakoff, A. 2015. "Real-time biopolitics: The actuary and the sentinel in global public health." *Economy and Society* 44 (1):40–59. doi: 10.1080/03085147.2014.983833.
Lin, L, E Savoia, F Agboola, and K Viswanath. 2014. "What have we learned about communication inequalities during the H1N1 pandemic: A systematic review of the literature." *BMC Public Health* 14 (1):484. doi: 10.1186/1471-2458-14-484.
Lupton, D. 1999. "Archetypes of infection: People with HIV/AIDS in the Australian press in the mid 1990s." *Sociology of Health and Illness* 21 (1):37–53.
MacDonald, L, G Cairns, K Angus, and M de Andrade. 2013. "Promotional communications for influenza vaccination: A systematic review." *Journal of Health Communication* 18 (12):1523–1549. doi: 10.1080/10810730.2013.840697.
Mairal, G. 2011. "The history and the narrative of risk in the media." *Health, Risk & Society* 13 (1):65–79.
Martin, E. 1994. *Flexible bodies: Tracking immunity in American culture from the days of polio to the age of AIDS*. Boston: Beacon Press.
Niemi, M, and V Pitkanen. 2017. "Gendered use of experts in the media: Analysis of the gender gap in Finnish news journalism." *Public Understanding of Science* 26 (3):355–368.
Petryna, A 2003. *Life exposed: Biological citizens after Chernobyl*. Princeton: Princeton University Press.
Rose, N. 2007. *The politics of life itself: Biomedicine, power and subjectivity in the twenty-first century*. Princeton: Princeton University Press.
Rubin, G, Y Finn, H Potts, and S Michie. 2015. "Who is sceptical about emerging public health threats? Results from 39 national surveys in the United Kingdom." *Public Health* 129 (12):1553–1562.
Seale, C. 2002. *Media and health*. London: Sage.
Shih, T, R Wijaya, and D Brossard. 2008. "Media coverage of public health epidemics: Linking framing and issue attention cycle toward an integrated theory of print news coverage of epidemics." *Mass Communication and Society* 11 (2):141–160.
Squire, C, M Davis, C Esin, M Andrews, B Harrison, L Hyden, and M Hyden. 2014. *What is narrative research?* London: Bloomsbury Academic.
Ungar, S. 2000. "Knowledge, ignorance and the popular culture: Climate change versus the ozone hole." *Public Understanding of Science* 9:297–312.
Ungar, Sheldon. 2008. "Global bird flu communication: Hot crisis and media reassurance." *Science Communication* 29 (4):472–497.
Wagner-Egger, P, A Bangerter, I Gilles, E Green, D Rigaud, F Krings, C Staerklé, and A Clémence. 2011. "Lay perceptions of collectives at the outbreak of the H1N1 epidemic: Heroes, villains and victims." *Public Understanding of Science* 20 (4):461–476. doi: 10.1177/0963662510393605.

Wald, P. 2008. *Contagious: Cultures, carriers, and the outbreak narrative.* Durham: Duke University Press.
Wilson, L. 2009. Melbourne the swine flu capital of the world. *The Australian.* Accessed October 16, 2015. http://www.theaustralian.com.au/news/melbourne-the-swine-flu-capital-of-the-world/story-e6frg6n6-1225724193107.

8
"The Boy Who Cried Wolf" and Other Post-Trust Stories

What a scare! What hysteria we've had! Like it was just the news and the media, it was such a petrifying thing and then, at the end of the day, I think every second person ended up with it anyway. That's my perception. (Cindy, Sydney, 20s, Lung disease)

You're supposed to call NHS 24 and you're supposed to speak to somebody rather than go [to the GP], which makes sense. But then I think, "Well, how can you diagnose somebody over the phone about that?" I don't know whether I trust that phone diagnosis system. (Mary, Glasgow, 30s, Pregnant in 2009)

In addition to the myriad challenges of shaping the public response, public health systems around the world faced the problem that the pandemic turned out to be mild for most people, despite early signs that it might have been serious. On May 11, the World Health Organization (WHO) posted a web notice that the H1N1 virus appeared to be leading to "very mild illness in otherwise healthy people," but that nations and individuals should be alert (2011, page 57). It was estimated that by August 6, 2010, 18,449 people worldwide had died with laboratory-confirmed infections (World Health Organization 2010). It was estimated in the United Kingdom that, as of March 18, 2010, 457 people had died (Hine 2010) and in Australia, by December 18, 2009, 191 people died (Australian Government Department of Health and Ageing 2009). As the pandemic ebbed away in 2010, Canada reported a total of 428 deaths (Eggleton and Ogilvie 2010), and Europe reported 1,975 (European Centre for Disease Prevention and Control 2010). Since 2010, however, epidemiologists have revised mortality estimates and have suggested that the global death rate may have been up to 10 times higher due to underreporting (Simonsen et al. 2013). Even so, the 2009 pandemic did not appear to lead to more deaths than normally associated with seasonal influenza, which is thought to be associated with between 250,000 and 500,000 deaths worldwide (World Health Organization 2014). It has also been estimated that the 2009 pandemic was more severe in the United States and Mexico than it was in Australia and the United Kingdom (Simonsen et al. 2013). The 2009 pandemic, therefore, was not the globalizing crisis it might have been, a feature of the event that became important to the governmental and social responses to this and possible future pandemics.

The pandemic, then, became something of a false alarm. Cindy's earlier comment reflected this idea and echoed the public view we discussed in the previous chapter that the news media had hyped the pandemic but also that this way of telling the pandemic story did not match the eventual mildness of the infection experienced by many people. As we have pointed out, the news media were found to have been mainly responsible reporters of facts and figures. Publics, however, identified news media as having circulated a story of global crisis, a perspective we attributed to the scale of reporting and the more general and familiar pandemic narrative. Cindy's use of "hysteria" was a way of emphasizing the contrast between what she saw as media hype and what actually happened. Cindy's account and others like it also reflected hindsight and in particular the standpoint of looking back on what had happened when it was accepted that the pandemic was, in general, mild. As we have noted in chapter 2, retrospective narration is not only a matter of casting over past events and reflecting on their meaning, it can also be a basis for self-understanding and, in particular, reflection on the moral virtues of one's actions and those of others (Freeman 2010). What has happened can shape one's view of the past, a perspective on experience that seems acutely salient for an unrealized global crisis like the 2009 pandemic. Cindy's reflections on hysteria shade into the realm of moral judgment on the basis of knowledge that what actually happened did not turn out to be a global crisis.

Implied, then, in Cindy's comment and foregrounded in Mary's was the challenge to public trust in the experts who decided what had to be done in 2009. Mary, who was introduced in chapter 3, expressed distrust in the telephone triage used to manage pandemic influenza in 2009. Seale et al. in Australia (2009) and Rubin et al. in the United Kingdom (2009) found that only minorities or slight majorities reported that they had adopted the hygiene and social distancing methods advocated by public health. Another indicator of the failure of trust is said to be the public response to vaccination. A 2009 survey of members of the general public in the Netherlands (van der Weerd et al. 2011) showed that lower levels of trust in public health advice were associated with lower intentions to take up the H1N1 vaccine. A UK survey showed that only 21.6% of pregnant women were vaccinated in 2009 (Sammon et al. 2013), though higher rates of vaccine uptake were reported for other groups at risk (40.3%), pregnant women with other diseases (33.1%), and pregnant women in Scotland (40%). In an audit of vaccination at Western Australian antenatal clinics, only 6.9% of eligible pregnant women were vaccinated (White, Petersen, and Quinlivan 2010). White et al., like Sammon et al., attributed this finding to concerns regarding the safety of the vaccine. Hilton and Smith, in their focus groups in Scotland, found that the pregnant women expressed anxiety with regard to vaccines with three of them referencing the side effects of thalidomide to justify their decision to not vaccinate (2010).

The eventual mildness of the pandemic also raised questions about the conduct of the WHO, in particular. The WHO emergency committee was singled out for criticism since some of its expert advisers were said to have had compromising links with pharmaceutical companies that benefited from national plans to stockpile antivirals (Cohen and Carter 2010, Flynn 2010, Godlee 2010). It is estimated that, worldwide, billions were spent on preparations for the pandemic. The United Kingdom was reported to have spent £1.2 billion, approximately, on the overall response including on vaccines, infrastructure, and communications (Hine 2010), and Australia spent AUD $200 million, the majority of which purchased the 21 million doses of the vaccine (Australian Broadcasting Corporation 2011). The WHO's and other national reviews were careful to not adopt a hypercritical stance, however. The United Kingdom's review (Hine 2010), stated that although it was possible to see that mistakes were made, criticism ought to be tempered with recognition that it was not possible to know ahead of time how the pandemic would evolve. In her foreword to the report, Dame Deidre Hine noted: "I am very aware of my responsibility to use hindsight sparingly" (2010, 2), underlining in another way the moral import of looking back on events in light of the present and what these reflections can mean for reputations and relationships into the future (Freeman 2010). Others have argued that, since the 2009 pandemic, building and sustaining trust will require efforts on the part of the public health system to enter into productive dialogue with publics, in place of what is seen as the tendency to adopt top-down communications approaches (Bangerter 2014). Against this background of what some have said was the false alarm of 2009, asking the general public to prepare themselves for another global public health emergency may face resistance and skepticism.

Arresting the apparent erosion of trust in pandemic preparedness and response has been the topic of some debate. A survey conducted in the United States in June and July 2009 (Freimuth et al. 2014) found that only a minority believed that the government could be trusted for its approach to the pandemic. Trust was operationalized as an aggregate of measures of the extent to which the government and its spokespersons were regarded as "committed," "caring and concerned," "open," "competent," "honest," "interested in citizens' best interest," and prepared to "act to protect citizens." The survey researchers attributed the observed weakness of trust in government to, among other factors, the notion that "communication has changed from top-down expert to consumer systems to non-hierarchical dialogue based systems" (2014, page 336). Similarly, a review of research on communications and communicable diseases (Cairns, de Andrade, and MacDonald 2013) has found that the promotion of trust lacks an evidence base but that the promotion of dialogue with affected publics and the credibility of the message provider may be significant factors. The editorial introduction of a special issue in the *European Psychologist* titled "Infectious Diseases Outbreaks and Public Trust" argued that to be effective in promoting and sustaining behavior change, public health communications need to engage with the "active sensemaking" of members of the general population (Bangerter 2014, page 3).

Deeply inscribed dynamics of power and inequality are also implicated in trust politics, a point made by Briggs and Briggs-Mantini (2003), Farmer (1999), and Singer (2016), among others. As Freimuth et al. (2014) noted, the patterns of trust in government they observed in their US population survey resonated with the long-standing marginalization of black and Hispanic people in healthcare and also memorable episodes of unethical practices in medicine, for example, the Tuskegee syphilis observational research from the 1930s. Trust relations are multifaceted and complexly interrelated, involving as they do the public institution of medicine, the organizations that constitute healthcare, biomedical knowledge systems, and related technologies (Calnan and Rowe 2008, Brown and Calnan 2015). Arresting the dissolution of trust in relation to pandemic communications, then, faces the challenge of long-standing and systemic forms of social exclusion and failures of trust.

Pandemic influenza, too, may have special status in relation to trust, since the 2009 pandemic was not the only false alarm associated with an H1N1 virus. As we discussed in chapter 2, the 1976 outbreak of H1N1 in the United

States also turned out to be less serious than first thought and therefore became a challenge to trust in public health systems (Fineberg 2008). Moreover, the attempt to vaccinate the entire population led to serious side effects and the cessation of the program. The resulting news media criticism was a major challenge to public health expertise and a lesson in communications in the context of uncertainties regarding how an influenza virus will behave. The events of 1976 and 2009, therefore, bear similarities and imply that the communication of public trust with regard to the management of pandemics has been a challenge for some time and that, as history would have it, H1N1 was the virus in question on both occasions. Because it ended up being a mild pandemic for most of those affected, the 2009 event has also been typified as the "pandemic that never was" in news reporting (Cresswell 2010), echoing the title of Fineberg and Neustadt's book on the 1976 pandemic, *The Epidemic That Never Was*.

These challenges of false alarm and trust are also connected with the precautionary principle and the related obligation to act in the face of uncertainty. As explained in chapter 1 influenza viruses have biological characteristics that make them radically uncertain, which means that presently it cannot be known before a pandemic occurs how severe it will actually be. In response to this uncertainty, pandemic preparedness plans adopt the precautionary principle. A webpage from the European regional office of the WHO was titled "The Precautionary Principle: Plan for the Worst, Hope for the Best" and explained the public health orientation to the potential of a false alarm in this way:

> When the WHO Director-General declared the pandemic, it met all the criteria of a pandemic. In the early stages of the event, it was impossible to know whether the pandemic would resemble the severe pandemic of 1918–19, or a much more mild pandemic. Initial indications coming out of Mexico were of a very severe event. While WHO elaborated various scenarios, including severe events, and spoke of these in its documents and on its web site, the world was fortunate in that the pandemic turned out to be moderate in its effects. This was made clear by the WHO Director-General in her statements during the course of the event. The exact death toll of the pandemic will never be known. Laboratory-confirmed deaths were 18,500, but this number under-states the true number of deaths. Moreover, severe disease and deaths did occur, with up to one third to half occurring in previously healthy young and middle-aged people. This coupled with the fact

that influenza viruses are unpredictable, supports the caution opted for by decision-makers and public health officials. The world used the precautionary principle to protect lives, which has to be part of any security plan (World Health Organization 2011b).

Because it was not, and still is not, easy to assess ahead of time how serious an outbreak will be, the WHO and many other public health authorities around the globe took the view in 2009 that: "in the face of uncertainty and potentially serious harm, it is better to err on the side of safety" (2011a, page 10). This prudent approach was couched in this way in Australia's governmental review of the 2009 response:

> While there were some signs indicating that the illness was moderate overall, Australia could not be complacent about the impact of the disease around the world and in Australia. This was a new virus, a new problem, and therefore initially, before we knew the clinical picture, we did not know what this new virus would do (Australian Government Department of Health and Ageing 2011, page 2).

The obligation to act in the face of uncertainty implies "manufactured uncertainties" (Beck 2009, page 291), in particular, that efforts to manage the risk of pandemic influenza produce other, subsidiary risks—such as false alarm—which feed back into the risk management approaches for pandemic influenza, complicating communications and potentially undoing efforts to reduce risk. The uncertainty of pandemic influenza, therefore, forces governments to take and make risks, imbuing communications on pandemics with a pervading, multilayered riskiness. As Hallin and Briggs explained (2015), the premediatization of pandemic communications may have engaged with this risk-producing potential of false alarm. "Be alert, not alarmed" can be seen as a method of reining in manufactured risk; it is a premediatization of false alarm, fashioned to sidestep the trust ramifications of outright false alarm, but flexible enough to be converted to alarm if the situation required it.

As we will see, however, the implied false alarm of the 2009 pandemic mobilized a narrative among our research participants that employed "The boy who cried wolf" fable and its compelling dramatization of the jeopardy faced by those who give a false impression of threat to life. Nerlich and Koteyko, in their textual analysis of United Kingdom news media and related blogs on H1N1, have identified the cry wolf "cliché," as they call it, as itself a feature of news media (2012). In this view, the problem of false alarm became a turn in the news storytelling on the pandemic, signaling troubles for the knowledge systems of public health in the United Kingdom and the communications they supported. This chapter, therefore, considers the talk of our respondents that explored the implications of loss of trust tied to the prospect of false alarm and offered other explanations for how people acted in the ways they said they had done in 2009.

"Crying Wolf"

As noted, communications and public health researchers have examined trust in connection with the 2009 pandemic (Bangerter 2014) and the more general ramifications of false alarm for efforts to manage infectious diseases and vaccination (Yaqub et al. 2014). The risks of false alarm were also well known to public health professionals in 2009. In related research of ours on the public policy response to pandemic influenza (Davis, Flowers, and Stephenson 2013), a health professional made this comment regarding public health communications:

> The challenge we had I think from a consumer point of view, if that's a right word, if we're summing up a lot of incidents or events in the last decade, Y2K, you know, we had September 11, and potential chemical, biological, terrorist type events, being on alarms and all that sort of stuff, we had our SARS. We have to be very careful that we don't have, "The boy who cried wolf," type syndrome as well because that does create apathy and resistance I guess. (Public health professional, 2009, Australia)

This quotation maps out some of the global crises that prefigured the 2009 pandemic, the related problem of false alarm and the potential for these events and effects to hamper efforts to shape public engagements with risk. It indicated a post-trust orientation to pandemic messaging in the sense that it recognized that the potential for the loss of trust was factored into communications on the 2009 pandemic. Notable in this quotation was the supposed complacency—"apathy and resistance"—on the part of the general public if alerts and warnings were used too often, underlined by reference to "The boy who cried wolf" fable. Reference to the fable has also been used by researchers to explain the communications challenge posed by the unfolding events of the 2009 pandemic and in particular the low death rate that quickly became apparent (Fogarty et al. 2011). Moreover, Holland and Blood's Australian respondents made reference to "cry wolf" in their reflections on the news media (2012). The folktale and its implications connect with what Joffe has referred to as "fatigue" on the part of the general public with regard to the repeated messages of the threat of emerging infectious diseases (2011).

These references to the "cried wolf" folktale underline the importance of narrative for engagements with the pandemic. The folktale is a highly codified and well-known moral story that dramatizes the social relations of trust and, in particular, its fragility and loss. The folktale is thought to have origins in classical, moral philosophy (Dorfman and Brewerm 1994) and teaches a lesson regarding the social consequences of lying. Telling lies, or misrepresenting reality, is thought to jeopardize the social standing of the person who "cries wolf" and even, in some versions of the fable, leads to their annihilation. Notably, the folktale works in two ways since it warns of the social consequences of lying but also points to the ramifications for collective responses to danger that arise through the repetition of false alarm. The folktale, like folktales in general, has a mythical, panhistoric quality that contributes to its forcefulness as an explanation of the loss of trust. It indicates also that after a certain point of repeated betrayal, trust is beyond repair. The folktale suggests therefore the importance of protecting trust as a method for securing cooperation, reducing harm, and promoting harmony, more generally. The folktale is of course exaggerated for narrative effect and is, perhaps, overused, but it nevertheless emerged as an important marker of what we refer to as the post-trust storytelling of the 2009 pandemic.

In a focus group of people living in Sydney with lung disease, reference was made to the "cry wolf" folktale in connection with messages regarding the 2009 pandemic. In what follows, several people in the focus group respond to a question on how they had heard of the pandemic:

BEATRICE: Public awareness campaigns on TV I think.
INTERVIEWER: On TV?
BEATRICE: I don't know—about masks and all that. We've become a nanny state, you know. [Beatrice says ironically] We think the government should give us everything, you know. [Interjection: Yeah, well] We've gotta do it for ourselves.
[Participants talk over each other]

BEATRICE: We need an intensive ad campaign for this winter, if it hits Europe or America, or something, then they're gonna step it up here and [Yeah] start telling us what we can expect next winter, and so on, and what we should be doing, and all the rest of it. And that's all you can do. [Yeah] You can't force people.

[Participants talk over each other]

HANNAH: You know there's so many things like global warming or this and that, or swine flu, all these things, we are likely to be threatened with, and the Y2K.

INTERVIEWER: Do you think maybe the media's hyping or making us more concerned with things like this?

HANNAH: Oh I think the media nearly always [Oh yeah] . . . that's why it's very hard to sort the information out at times.

PAULINE: I have found that trying to sort out information, yes, but when they've had things like the swine flu, pandemics of any sort overseas, Asian countries and so forth. Okay, have we got it here or have we got it there, or what are they doing about it?

BEATRICE: It's got to the stage where if you work out over the last 15 years and you start thinking about all the things that we've supposedly been panicked about, every couple of years when we get ho-hum about one, another one comes up. [Yeah, no, it's true] Like the Y2K thing; nothing happened. Somebody made a heap of money out of it and you get the flu thing that big panic, nothing happened. Now we've got global warming and what-not. That's all over. Nothing happened.

HANNAH: Anything can happen anywhere. [But it's not likely] [You've just gotta be on your toes] They won't be happy here 'til there's terrorists. Look at all that's happened.

BOB: God, that could happen anytime here too.

HANNAH: Yeah, but how likely, really? Anything can. [Yeah] You get those television things and somebody, I don't know, swallows a frog in Japan or something and they say, "Could this happen in Australia?" [Yeah, of course it could] It just drives you mad. [Yeah]

INTERVIEWER: Yeah, well I guess it's the speculation.

SUZANNE: I canceled the papers. I thought, "What's the point?"

BEATRICE: Yeah, but it's like the boy who cried wolf: they try and scare you every couple of years with something and then we just say, "Oh yeah, this is another one," because they've all fizzed out.

SUZANNE: It's all garbage. (Sydney Focus Group, 50s to 60s, Lung disease)

The consensus built in this passage was that the repeated message of the dangers of pandemics and other threats reduced the believability of the threat and those who seek to perpetuate it. "Fizzed out" and "garbage" signified what appeared to be active rejection of the pandemic message, even among a group of people with lung disease and therefore likely to be at heightened risk. Importantly, however, the news media was the focus of this criticism, as we discussed in the previous chapter. Beatrice in particular made mention of "the boy who cried wolf" and associated skepticism with regard to her reception of news media. The figure of the public health expert evaded criticism, perhaps due to the ways in which health communications may have, in the mode of premediatization, furthered the idea of the public health expert as the authoritative, fact provider in the pandemic story. Notable too was Beatrice's reference to the "nanny state" and therefore the importance of self-reliance on the part of ordinary citizens.

Other research participants spoke of the notion of false alarm and its implications. Peter, from Melbourne and introduced in chapter 7, made this comment in response to a question from the interviewer regarding the cost of the public health response to the pandemic in 2009:

> [It's a] wasteful thing that the government does. And a knee-jerk reaction by the government again. Spend money that's not theirs. And when there is no real need for it. So again that would make you a little bit more skeptical the next time something's happened. And this is where problems can arise in the future because we don't believe our government is responsible enough to make the wise decisions and the right decision when the time comes. So in the future I can see if there is a pandemic, something deadly, something really bad, a lot of people are going to get very hurt and very sick, and/or die because of the lack of trust we have in our government. Because of the decisions they made in the past. (Peter, Melbourne, 50s, No disclosed health problems)

Peter demonstrated awareness, then, of the lesson of the "cried wolf" folktale and, like the public health professional and Beatrice from the focus group, could foresee troubles for the management of future pandemics. His account suggested a degree of skepticism attached to the news media surrounding the 2009 pandemic but also in relation to global threats more generally. His point of view marks the post-trust context into which messages of new threats are digested and understood. Marilyn, who lived in Melbourne and was pregnant in 2009, was asked to comment on how the mildness of the 2009 pandemic might influence public responses to future ones. Her account indicated that it was important to protect trust because of the potential severity of a pandemic event:

> I think it's a worry. But I think, see you have to trust your governments. Whether you like them or approve of their politics, or anything like that, you have to be able to trust them. And you trust that they're going to look after you—not just, I mean financially and all that sort of thing. I don't mean Big Brother looking over your shoulder—but that's their job. If something like that [pandemic] comes along, it's up to them, with their experts as I said before, their advisors, expert advisors in the medical fields and all that, to tell them what to expect and what could happen if they didn't do A, B and C. And you'd hope that they would do A, B and C, and maybe save our lives. Save the community. That's their job. I think people are very skeptical of their governments but I think that's irrelevant. It doesn't seem to affect governments: they still tend to meddle and, and do things [people] don't like. But I still think that that's what they've gotta do. That's what they have to do and if there's any doubt about anything, they've gotta act. 'Cause their advisors will advise them that way. (Marilyn, Melbourne, 30s, Pregnant in 2009)

Where Beatrice and her colleagues had spoken of the loss of trust and Peter reflected on its value for intervention in future pandemics, Marilyn implied that publics were bound to trust their governments, regardless of their skepticism and, by implication, distrust. She implied that a genuine threat would have to be faced by government, which meant that, individuals would therefore have no choice but to comply with experts and officials. This way of talking about trust captured something of the situation all would face in the event of a catastrophe. A future, severe pandemic would require all to rely on their governments as a matter of survival. Her account, too, made reference to "expert advisors" who could be relied on to shape what governments did. In this account, experts and their knowledge become trustworthy, and necessarily so, despite skepticism with regard to government in general, echoing or perhaps reiterating the way the news media texts appeared to have established the hero role of the public health professional in the pandemic drama.

Another version of "cry wolf" storytelling was apparent in Cameron's interview in response to a question on his news media engagement in 2009.

Cameron was introduced in chapter 1 through his infection story. Like the people in the focus group discussed earlier, Cameron was rather skeptical, though playfully so:

INTERVIEWER: Yeah, the newspapers, the TV, what do you remember from that time?
CAMERON: "Oh here we go!" That's how I felt, you know we're going to have this for bloody months, we're going to have this for ages and I just think it's just everywhere you know the whole, it's like a band wagon, or the gravy train and you know they're all jumping on it and it's like big news at the moment and when one bad thing happens and say in sort of the social services you know, "The social services they're all evil they don't do their job right" and it's like, "Oh, I've got another story about that and we'll pump out another story about that and oh, I've got another one and another one" and these things are happening all the time and you know it's like I can remember . . . oh, it wasn't long after the first time I was in India, somebody has got the plague in the UK. The plague is in India all the time, it never went away! "Oh, we need to spray all the planes!" The plague is there all the time! Well it ebbs and flows, especially in cities and stuff. You know, but it's like one case of it and then (mock panic) "Waaaaaah! Let's run down the streets screaming with no clothes on!" or something you know, covered in burning tar (laughs) or something! That's what it's like though, it's awful. (laughs) (Cameron, Glasgow, 40s, No disclosed health problems)

Cameron created an amusing picture of media frenzy on the pandemic and indirectly made reference to the inadequacies of the National Health Service, a theme that emerged in research in the United Kingdom on general public narrative on Methicillin-resistant Staphylococcus aureus (MRSA) (Joffe, Washer, and Solberg 2011, Washer and Joffe 2006, Washer, Joffe, and Solberg 2008). His account showed an assumption of the self-interested nature of the news media, which for him had repeated the "plague" message far too often and played to xenophobic ideas of disease and its origins. This extract implied that Cameron colored his account with nonverbal "mock panic," underlining how the news media had hyped the story and therefore accentuated the sense of false alarm. Cameron, however, like many of our respondents, misrepresented the actual content of the news media texts in 2009. It appeared that, despite the predominance of facts in news reporting and a general message of "Be alert, not alarmed," the message of hype and the linked message of false alarm had taken hold for Cameron, accentuating the doubting public reception of communications on the threat posed by the pandemic.

It also appeared to be the case that hype—in actuality or by reputation—led some of our research participants to turn away from news media, another ripple in the biopolitics of trust. In Liz and Peter's interview, the interviewer noted that some schools in Melbourne had been closed during the pandemic. Liz and Peter, who were introduced in the previous chapter, found this information disconcerting and, because they had missed it at the time, debated together whether the "government" had acted strongly enough to inform its citizenry:

PETER: Was it as widespread as we were meant to believe? Because we would hear instances in the press, but not widespread instances. So we became skeptics. Was the government not doing enough to let us know what the real danger was? Not just press reports, you know, a two-minute grab on the six o'clock news or a three-paragraph something in page seven of the local paper, The Herald Sun [tabloid newspaper]. If it was as bad as what I'm thinking now where they're closing down schools, should it have been made some sort of proclamation in full page ads by the press, by the government of the day? And I can't remember that happening.
INTERVIEWER: Are you saying that you think that that should have happened?
PETER: If it was as bad as the questions you're asking me are leading me to think then yes it should have happened. They should have made it more urgent, I s'pose and for our attention, that this is happening. Giving us the facts. They might not have wanted to panic us but, in the meantime, we went the other way where we didn't think about it at all. (Peter, Melbourne, 50s, No disclosed health problems)

Peter, like other people in our interviews and focus groups, showed some awareness of the "Be alert, not alarmed" logic of health communications and the related effort to avoid panicking his fellow citizens. He signaled though that he and Liz had adopted the position of skeptics or, in other terms, had afforded themselves a kind of immunity from what they, like many others, saw as news media hype. He was also adamant that the news media were therefore not the right vehicle for informing him of the seriousness of the pandemic. Liz and Peter suggested that a direct link with the public health system and therefore one that circumvented the news may have been more appropriate for them:

LIZ: I was told that there was a pandemic. Yes, it was very serious, but I still wasn't concerned. So it wasn't so much the lack of knowledge that there was one. It's for whatever reason in my world I was okay. If it was worse than that we should be then warned on a daily basis, should have been a letter drop about it. But obviously if there isn't a huge warning about it, you're not so concerned. So, you know, it's every individual's responsibility to look after themselves, too.

PETER: Yeah. I'm just saying that if it's only reporting on it, you don't take it with as much fact or credence [Liz: Authority] as if we actually get a notification like a page ad and saying, "This is what is happening. This is from your government. This is from your medical doctors, etc., stating that this will happen, blah, blah, blah." Instead of just these little grabs here and there. And it's always panic, someone else has got it, you know, someone's sick of it. I don't think they had a constructive way of informing us.

Liz, picking up on Peter's argument, suggested that public health experts ought to send their message in the form of a letter drop to connect citizens more directly with government or, more particularly, with public health experts. In the United Kingdom in 2009, an information booklet was delivered to every household as part of the pandemic communications strategy launched on April 30 (Hine 2010). The booklet featured the "sneezing man" on its cover. Direct-to-household communication was not adopted in Australia in 2009 (Australian Government Department of Health and Ageing 2011). This method of direct instruction is perhaps seen to be outside of the hype that troubles other pandemic messages, though it is of course a communications strategy that faces other risks. Previously we commented that the shape of the news media on the pandemic—its sheer scale, shape, and repetition of facts pertaining to the progress and retreat of the pandemic—was itself a message for publics. It may then also be the case that giving a leaflet to householders may carry some symbolic weight, even in, or perhaps because of, the present age of hypermediated social relations and the travels of pandemic narrative across media. Peter, too, seemed to suggest that a trustworthy message was required in part because of the news media context within which most people received information on the pandemic. As

Liz pointed out, however, citizens in her estimation should also be expected to act for themselves and not depend on government to tell them what to do. The adoption of direct communications also reduces the benefit of using the diversity and power of news media to amplify and circulate the message of pandemic preparedness. Relatedly, though, going outside of the news media to reach publics also runs the risk that public health authorities may then themselves face the biopolitics of false alarm, which, as we have indicated, seems to focus on news media representations and not the authority of expert knowledge. Is the news media and its reputation for hype, then, an important way for public health systems to deflect loss of trust and false alarm? This perspective is another way in which the form of communications is more important than what content is transmitted. Publics and the public health system blame the messenger, perhaps a convenient organization of communications for the post-trust era.

Vaccination

Our research participants also shed some light on the observations of poor uptake of the vaccine in 2009. As we noted in chapter 2, fewer than one in five (20/116) people in our research reported having been vaccinated in 2009, though recall of the dates and types of vaccination was in general hazy among people in our research. In contrast, a slight majority (64/116) reported that they had been vaccinated at any time in their lives. This high proportion may have reflected the bias in our sampling toward people with specific vulnerabilities for pandemic influenza, in particular: nearly all of the older people (8/10) and people with immune and respiratory illness (39/44) reported any lifetime vaccination. One in five (11/47) people from our "healthy" group and two in five (6/15) of the pregnant women reported any vaccination. These lower proportions may reflect the relative health of these groups, though we hasten to add that it is not feasible to make inferences about vaccination behavior based on our samples of volunteers.

Perhaps because so many had vaccinated in their lifetimes, people in our interviews and focus groups did not speak against vaccination technology in a strident manner and, despite the events of 2009, retained trust in biomedical powers. But questions and doubts were expressed. Marie, from Sydney and in the "healthy" group, as noted in chapter 6, indicated that the vaccine promoted in 2009 was untested:

INTERVIEWER: What did you think of like the Australian government's response to the threat of pandemic influenza in 2009?
MARIE: I like how they had a vaccination all sorted out in a heartbeat. That I don't trust.
INTERVIEWER: Why don't you trust it?
MARIE: Because it doesn't give it time to figure out what's wrong with it. . . . And you sit there and go . . . but it's not tested. There's no long-term test to it so everybody gets it but, in the long run, what's gonna happen? (Sydney, 20s, No disclosed health problems)

In contrast, Vaughn, also from the "healthy" group in Sydney, expressed belief in biomedicine. He said that he would use an influenza vaccine, though he also seemed to conflate vaccine technology and treatment:

INTERVIEWER: In general, do you have a trust of science? I mean you indicated that the vaccine . . .
VAUGHN: I definitely have a trust of science. I think I'm also lazy when it comes to vaccines. It's not necessarily that I distrust them or that other people should or shouldn't take them. Individual choice is what we have here, that's what we're gifted with and like I'll take it if I get sick. (Sydney, 20s, No disclosed health problems)

Vaughn captured the sense in which our participants held onto the idea that medicine could be trusted to control disease. While there was much criticism of media hype and awareness of the drawbacks of false alarm, medicine itself was spoken of as a constant and trustworthy benefit of life in affluent countries. This core trust in medicine also seemed to be an imperative for those with health problems. Cindy, whose commentary introduced this chapter, said, "I've got trust in the experts and if they say it's AOK then I'm happy to swallow whatever they want me to" (Sydney, 20s, lung disease). Cindy implied that she had to trust in medicine because her health depended on it. Trust in this context therefore had ramifications for a secure sense of being able to survive serious illness and relatedly, being in the world, or ontological security of self (Giddens 1990). Marilyn, first discussed in chapter 6, argued that her trust in medicine and its practitioners was needed as she did not have sufficient knowledge of her own:

I don't know anything about them [vaccines and antivirals]. I just put a lot of trust in my doctor. I mean he always advises me to do the right thing but otherwise I don't know much about them at all. So really, when it comes down to it, I've got a lot of trust in my doctor. (Melbourne, 30s, Pregnant in 2009)

These extracts reveal the manifold challenges and ramifications of trust: doubt with regard to the scientific practices and judgments that underpin the use of vaccines in time of a pandemic threat (Marie), a self-confessed "lazy" trust that vaccines will protect health (Vaughan), trust as a matter of survival and perhaps ontological security (Cindy), and trust as a solution to lack of personal expertise (Marilyn). These engagements with trust were thrown into sharp relief by some of the pregnant women in our research who did report that they had concerns in 2009 regarding vaccination. Linda from Sydney and pregnant in 2009, was not certain if she would vaccinate her child for influenza:

I don't know. Maybe. He might be a bit . . . I think this year maybe. He doesn't breathe very well through his nose. He's a mouth breather and he had surgery to remove his adenoids a few months ago. So maybe he might be a bit more prone to things 'cause his breathing is not so good and he's had surgery, so maybe his immunity's a bit low . . . so maybe. Maybe I might get it for him next year.
Interviewer: Bit of a hard decision, isn't it?
Linda: See how he is. I don't really trust the medical profession when they say things are safe or not safe. (Sydney, 30s, Pregnant in 2009)

Linda depicted herself as undecided and linked this position with distrust of medical practitioners and in particular their estimation of the safety of medical technologies. Her consideration of vaccines was also laced together with information regarding the health situation of her child, a perspective she elaborated on later in her interview when asked to comment on the 2009 vaccine:

INTERVIEWER: So the media hype around the time didn't influence your decisions in any way to like have the vaccine or things like that?
LINDA: No. I just rang them and found out. I talked to the doctors. But again, I don't trust doctors or they always just take the option of whatever their books say is the safest, most conservative option. I don't trust them at all. I mean when my baby was born, the pediatricians in the hospital . . . it was like the dark ages. His breathing was a bit funny. So they put him on

oxygen straight away. I wanted to just go home. I was planning to have a home birth but I was in labor for three days so went in and got some drugs to make the baby come. Which was good: I was happy to use the hospital when I needed them. Then I wanted to go home. They're just so paranoid and do everything for the sake of what they call "safety."

Linda reiterated what she identified as a lack of trust through the story of her son's birth and care in the hospital. She did not express outright dismissal of medicine but gave the impression that she was cautious and selective. When pressed on the reasons why she chose childhood vaccinations for her son, Linda indicated, like Marilyn earlier, that fully fledged engagement with the expert knowledge on vaccination and risk was beyond her:

LINDA: I can see that they [vaccines] have changed, you know, we used to have various diseases and now we don't. So I bet they do in third world countries. I don't know what they are. TB and stuff like that. As I say, that's one of the reasons that I decided to get him [son] vaccinated was because I wasn't prepared to look into it enough to make an informed decision. It's pretty hard.
INTERVIEWER: What would be an informed decision for you?
LINDA: I'd wanna look at a fair bit of literature. But when you look at a lot of it, both sides are pretty, like the anti-vaccine people, they seem quite a bit rabid and . . . I wasn't trusting them either.

Linda therefore indicated reliance on vaccine technology despite her more general distrust of medicine. This reluctant "trust by default" was also in counterpoint to the position of the antivaxers, which was not to be trusted, either. Linda therefore created a narrative of conflictual engagements with trust, expert knowledge, and vaccine technology. It appeared, then, that parents like Linda did not then simply face questions of the safety or not of vaccines, but contended with the multiple currents and tensions on the value and risks of vaccines. Similarly, Rebecca, who was introduced in chapter 3, spoke of resisting the distrust narrative as she prepared for the birth of her child:

When I was pregnant and I would go to (laughs) I used to go along to these birth preparation classes and yoga classes and these birthing classes and they were really nice. The yoga classes were brilliant and you'd have an hour or so of yoga and it was really good and then at the end they would chat to you about birth and talk to you all about all the different types of birth you could have and blah, blah, blah. (pause) I discounted the yoga entirely because they'd spend the whole time saying, "The medics are all out to get you," and, "They'll force you to do this and they'll drag the baby out kicking and screaming and they'll do everything," like this and they were so antimedicine and anti-NHS and antidoctors and antimidwives, and everybody was, "Go in ready for a fight because you're going to get one!," and I never once felt like I was having a fight with anybody! But I can quite imagine that group would've had a field day with this vaccination! (laughs) I have trust in the medical profession and I suppose that a lot of other people are wary and have concerns about the medical profession and maybe I'm too naïve about it and I need to be a bit more conservative with my opinions. (Glasgow, 30s, Pregnant in 2009)

The story that Rebecca provided of her yoga friends underlined the sense in which she and Linda were caught at the intersection of competing claims on the trustworthiness of medicine. The problem of trust, which concerned pandemic communications and in particular the promotion of vaccination, was therefore articulated with the more general dynamics of pregnancy and medicine (Katz Rothman 2007). This is an important connection: pandemic communications need to be sensitive to the lives that expectant mothers lead and the dilemmas of expert knowledge, trust, and risk they are compelled to negotiate. Claire, who was first introduced in chapter 4, also spoke of the challenges of engaging with the healthcare system in relation to vaccination in 2009:

Well it was so difficult just trying to get information and I was just so confused what to do because I got a letter from the GP inviting me to go. And I went and I said, "I don't know what to do because I'm not sure. I just want to talk about it, talk this over. I'm having a baby and I'm really confused." I felt pressurized to have it. It was quite, what's the word, judgmental? The GP said, "People like me are vulnerable, [which I'm not compared to a lot of people] and it was my responsibility to protect my unborn child from swine flu." But as a parent you think, "Oh my God!" But then the media was telling you people had had the vaccine and died after it or they'd had a really bad reaction. I don't think it was his comment, as the media was making that out. But there was a bit of scaremongering about the swine flu vaccination, but equally there were people actually dying of the swine flu. So it was like, "What the hell do you do?!" (laughs) It's like, "I'm pregnant I need to try and do what's best for my child." But the information I was getting was so judgmental, well as I found it. If I hadn't have agreed to that vaccination I would have felt hellish, like I had been a bad mother (laughs) or not been responsible. But I was really scared about getting it because of the stories I had heard in the media. But I wasn't getting any reassurance, if you like, that this would be like safe. So it was a difficult decision. (Glasgow, 30s, Pregnant in 2009)

Claire expressed some anxiety about the vaccine and depicted herself as caught between a medical imperative to act, a normative expectation of good motherhood, and stories in the news media that had said that the vaccine was dangerous. Claire's story was one of distrust, both of the medical system and the news media. In the end, it seemed that the social cost of not vaccinating—of jeopardizing her sense of herself as a good mother—was the most powerful force in her decision to vaccinate. Echoing Linda and Claire, Rebecca commented on how the expectation to vaccinate was complicated by her pregnancy and care of her other child:

I was pregnant so I had the swine flu vac myself and I also got [Rebecca's child] vaccinated because they were offering it for all children under five at the time. So we opted to have him vaccinated as well. Especially for me, thinking about why I had it for myself, and the baby, I was vaccinating myself for the baby.
[later]
(sigh) When you're pregnant it just becomes, everything just becomes about the baby. Everything you eat, everything you do, how much sleep you get, everything is for your baby, you just want to try and make your baby as healthy as possible and you want to try and keep your baby safe and so I just kept thinking, "If I get unwell, if something happens to me, if I get really ill then that's going to affect the baby and the baby is going to end up ill or . . . or worse" and I just couldn't you know. You just feel completely responsible you just feel like your whole everything, your whole life is for the baby.

Rebecca rather dramatically outlined how pregnancy and the advent of the pandemic coalesced in her life to foreground the profound ways in which mothering was subject to social norms of responsibility. In another context we have written about this aspect of our research and made links with feminist scholarship on pregnancy and motherhood (Lohm et al. 2014). Linda, Claire, and Rebecca suggested that trust in vaccine technology did figure in the reasons why some pregnant women did not readily choose to vaccinate in 2009 tied to their particular circumstances and also that those who did vaccinate did not find this action to be without consequences for their sense of personal security and well-being.

Pandemic communications, then, are also trust communications. Persuading publics that they might be at risk and should take action asks them to place trust in experts, their knowledge, and in public health more generally. The public reception of news media on the pandemic as hyped and the related idea of the public health expert as the voice of reason and calm is implicated in trust and its biopolitical ramifications for individuals. We have argued, too, that all the stories we have discussed are already after trust. The "cried wolf" folktale, for example, which informed the storytelling of people in our research and others in the field, indicated that before their inception pandemic communications and the news were open to questions and troubles of trust and distrust. As Hardin has argued, politics in general is enacted post-trust since a time or setting when trust was not a problem is a halcyon dream (2006).

This chapter has also shown that it is mistaken to assume that the subject of trust politics is universal. Trust and distrust articulate into the social worlds of pregnant women, men and women with chronic illness, and those who do not expect to become seriously ill with pandemic influenza, to name a few among many other life situations. As the accounts discussed in this chapter indicate, knowing which information and advice were trustworthy (Camporesi, Vaccarella, and Davis 2017), juggling what were at times competing notions of trust, and myriad practical considerations and, for pregnant women in our research, the confluence of motherhood and pandemic risk, mediated how individuals responded to the pandemic message.

References

Australian Broadcasting Corporation. 2011. "$200 million spend on swine flu pandemic." accessed October 13, 2015. http://www.abc.net.au/news/2011-01-08/200-million-spent-on-swine-flu-pandemic/1898184.

Australian Government Department of Health and Ageing. 2009. "Australian influenza surveillance summary report, No.32, 2009." Accessed October 7, 2015. http://www.health.gov.au/internet/main/publishing.nsf/Content/cda-ozflu-no32-09.htm.

Australian Government Department of Health and Ageing. 2011. *Review of Australia's health sector response to pandemic (H1N1) 2009: Lessons identified*. Canberra: Commonwealth of Australia.
Bangerter, A. 2014. "Investigating and rebuilding public trust in preparation for the next pandemic." *European Psychologist* 19 (1):1–3.
Beck, U. 2009. "World risk society and manufactured uncertainties." *Iris* 1 (2):291–299.
Briggs, C, and C Mantini-Briggs. 2003. *Stories in the time of cholera: Racial profiling during a medical nightmare*. Berkeley: University of California Press.
Brown, P, and M Calnan. 2015. "Chains of (dis)trust: Exploring the underpinnings of knowledge-sharing and quality care across mental health services." *Sociology of Health & Illness* 38 (2):286–305.
Cairns, G, M de Andrade, and L MacDonald. 2013. "Reputation, relationships, risk communication, and the role of trust in the prevention and control of communicable disease: A review." *Journal of Health Communication* 18 (12):1550–1565. doi: 10.1080/10810730.2013.840696.
Calnan, M, and R Rowe. 2008. *Trust matters in health care*. Maidenhead: McGaw-Hill.
Camporesi, S, M Vaccarella, and M Davis. 2017. "Investigating public trust in expert knowledge: Narrative, ethics, and engagement." In "Symposium: Public trust in expert knowledge." *Journal of Bioethical Inquiry* 14 (1):23–30. doi 10.1007/s11673-016-9767-4.
Cohen, D, and P Carter. 2010. "WHO and the pandemic flu 'conspiracies.'" *BMJ* 340:c2912.
Cresswell, A. 2010. "The pandemic that never was." *The Australian*. Accessed October 8, 2015. http://www.theaustralian.com.au/news/inquirer/the-pandemic-that-never-was/story-e6frg6z6-1225905590249.
Davis, M, P Flowers, and N Stephenson. 2013. "'We had to do what we thought was right at the time': Retrospective discourse on the 2009 H1N1 pandemic in the UK." *Sociology of Health & Illness* 36 (3):369–382.
Dorfman, M, and W Brewerm. 1994. "Understanding the points of fables." *Discourse Processes* 17:105–129.
Eggleton, A, and K Ogilvie. 2010. *Canada's response to the 2009 H1N1 influenza pandemic*. Ottawa: Standing Senate Committee on Social Affairs, Science and Technology.
European Centre for Disease Prevention and Control. 2010. *The 2009 A(H1N1) pandemic in Europe*. Stockholm: ECDC.
Farmer, P. 1999. *Infections and inequalities: The modern plagues*. Berkeley: University of California Press.
Fineberg, H. 2008. "Preparing for avian influenza: lessons from the 'swine flu affair.'" *Journal of Infectious Diseases* 197 (Suppl 1):S14–S18.
Flynn, P. 2010. "The handling of the H1N1 pandemic: more transparency needed." Parliamentary Assembly, Council of Europe. Online document. Accessed January 18, 2012. http://assembly.coe.int/CommitteeDocs/2010/20100604_H1n1pandemic_E.pdf.
Fogarty, A, K Holland, M Imison, R Blodd, S Chapman, and S Holding. 2011. "Communicating uncertainty—how Australian television reported H1N1 risk in 2009: A content analysis." *BMC Public Health* 11 (181).
Freeman, M. 2010. *Hindsight: The promise and peril of looking backward*. Oxford: Oxford University Press.
Freimuth, V, D Musa, K Hilyard, S Quinn, and K Kim. 2014. "Trust during the early stages of the 2009 H1N1 pandemic." *Journal of Health Communication* 19 (3):321–339. doi: 10.1080/10810730.2013.811323.
Giddens, A. 1990. *The consequences of modernity*. Cambridge: Polity.
Godlee, Fiona. 2010. "Conflicts of interest and pandemic flu." *BMJ* 340:c2947.

Hallin, DC, and CL Briggs. 2015. "Transcending the medical/media opposition in research on news coverage of health and medicine." *Media, Culture & Society* 37 (1):85–100. doi: 10.1177/0163443714549090.

Hardin, R. 2006. *Trust*. Cambridge: Polity.

Hilton, S, and E Smith. 2010. "Public views of the UK media and government reaction to the 2009 swine flu pandemic." *BMC Public Health* 10:697.

Hine, D. 2010. *The 2009 influenza pandemic: An independent review of the UK response to the 2009 influenza pandemic*. London: Pandemic Flu Response Review Team, Cabinet Office.

Holland, K, and W Blood. 2012. "Public responses and reflexivity during the swine flu pandemic in Australia." *Journalism Studies* 14 (4):523–538. iFirst: doi:10.1080/1461670X.2012.744552.

Joffe, H. 2011. "Public apprehension of emerging infectious diseases: Are changes afoot?" *Public Understanding of Science* 20 (4):446–460.

Joffe, H, P Washer, and C Solberg. 2011. "Public engagement with emerging infectious disease: The case of MRSA in Britain." *Psychology and Health* 26 (6):667–683.

Katz Rothman, B. 2007. "Introduction. A lifetime's labour: Women and power in the birthplace." In *Labouring on: Birth in transition in the United States (perspectives on gender)*, edited by W Simonds, B Katz Rothman, and B Norman, xi–xxii. New York: Routledge.

Lohm, D, P Flowers, N Stephenson, E Waller, and M Davis. 2014. "Biography, pandemic time and risk: Pregnant women reflecting on their experiences of the 2009 influenza pandemic." *Health: An Interdisciplinary Journal for the Social Study of Health, Illness and Medicine* 18 (5):493–508. 1363459313516135, first published on January 29, 2014.

Nerlich, B, and N Koteyko. 2012. "Crying wolf? Biosecurity and metacommunication in the context of the 2009 swine flu pandemic." *Health & Place* 18 (4):710–717. doi: http://dx.doi.org/10.1016/j.healthplace.2011.02.008.

Rubin, G, R Amlot, L Page, and S Wessely. 2009. "Public perceptions, anxiety, and behaviour change in relation to the swine flu outbreak: Cross sectional telephone survey." *British Medical Journal* 339:b2651.

Sammon, C, A McGrogan, J Snowball, and C de Vries. 2013. "Pandemic influenza vaccination during pregnancy: An investigation of vaccine uptake during the 2009/10 pandemic vaccination campaign in Great Britain." *Human Vaccines & Immunotherapeutics* 9 (4):917–923.

Seale, H, M McLaws, A Heywood, K Ward, C Lowbridge, D Van, J Gralton, and C MacIntyre. 2009. "The community's attitude towards swine flu and pandemic influenza." *Medical Journal of Australia* 191 (5):267–269.

Simonsen, L, P Spreeuwenberg, R Lustig, R Taylor, D Fleming, M Kroneman, M Van Kerkhove, A Mounts, J John Paget, and GLaMOR Collaborating Teams. 2013. "Global mortality estimates for the 2009 influenza pandemic from the GLaMOR project: A modeling study." *PLOS Medicine* 10 (11):e1001558.

Singer, M. 2016. "The spread of Zika and the potential for global arbovirus syndemics." *Global Public Health* 12 (1):1–18. doi: 10.1080/17441692.2016.1225112.

van der Weerd, W, D Timmermans, D Beaujean, J Oudhoff, and J van Steenbergen. 2011. "Monitoring the level of government trust, risk perception and intention of the general public to adopt protective measures during the influenza A (H1N1) pandemic in the Netherlands." *BMC Public Health* 19 (11):575.

Washer, P, and H Joffe. 2006. "The 'hospital superbug': Social representations of MRSA." *Social Science & Medicine* 63 (8):2141–2152. doi: http://dx.doi.org/10.1016/j.socscimed.2006.05.018.

Washer, P, H Joffe, and C Solberg. 2008. "Audience readings of media messages about MRSA." *Journal of Hospital Infection* 70 (1):42–47. doi: http://dx.doi.org/10.1016/j.jhin.2008.05.013.

White, S, R Petersen, and J Quinlivan. 2010. "Pandemic (H1N1) 2009 influenza vaccine uptake in pregnant women entering the 2010 influenza season in Western Australia." *MJA* 193:405–407.

World Health Organization (WHO). 2010. "Pandemic (H1N1) 2009—update 112." World Health Organization. Accessed July 7, 2011. http://www.who.int/csr/don/2010_08_06/en/index.html

World Health Organization (WHO). 2011a. *Implementation of the international health regulations (2005). Report of the Review Committee on the Functioning of the International Health Regulations (2005) in relation to Pandemic (H1N1) 2009. Report by the Director-General.* Geneva: World Health Organization.

World Health Organization (WHO). 2011b. "The precautionary principle: Plan for the worst, hope for the best." Accessed November 28. 2015. http://www.euro.who.int/en/health-topics/communicable-diseases/influenza/news/news/2011/11/who-response-to-concerns-in-serbia-over-its-actions-during-the-influenza-a-h1n1-2009-pandemic/the-precautionary-principle-plan-for-the-worst,-hope-for-the-best.

World Health Organization (WHO). 2014. "Influenza (seasonal) fact sheet No 211." March 2014. Accessed October 7, 2015. http://www.who.int/mediacentre/factsheets/fs211/en/.

Yaqub, O, S Castle-Clarke, N Sevdalis, and J Chataway. 2014. "Attitudes to vaccination: A critical review." *Social Science & Medicine* 112:1–11. doi: 10.1016/j.socscimed.2014.04.018.

9
Conclusion

Our book has considered the ways in which pandemic narratives and their metaphors travel across the media technologies of science and popular culture and into lived experience. As others have noted, personal stories on the 2009 pandemic (Hilton and Hunt 2011) and of previous ones (Belling 2009), are few and far between. The accounts we have produced in this book, then, have salience in and of themselves, but also for what they imply for communications on a global health threat and for the coming into being of useful narrative public health approaches.

Our analysis placed engagements with pandemic storytelling across public life in dialogue with the narratives on the enactment of expert advice. This dual approach helped to establish perspectives on how narratives influence publics to take action, or not. We took the view that narrative does not simply mediate pandemic knowledge and advice by helping to structure it intelligibly and meaningfully. We also questioned the idea that narratives persuade in and of themselves in ways that are not very far removed from now discredited notions of linear, hypodermic communications on matters of health. We adopted the view that media are thoroughly entangled with experience and that pandemic narratives found there help to constitute subjects and the relationships they have with the expert knowledge systems that underpin public health efforts to manage microbial threats. We drew on ideas of pandemic narrative culture (Wald 2008), biocommunicability (Briggs and Nichter 2009), and biological citizenship (Petersen et al. 2010) to explore biopolitical rationalities that pervade how experts and publics address themselves to a global health threat. Drawing on the idea of the narrator-listener relationship (Squire et al. 2014) and the related idea that narratives extract some of their effects in their reading, we explored the interpretation skills that individuals brought into their address to pandemic story-telling and how they spoke of appropriating, interpreting, refashioning, and resisting expert advice in the social settings they were required to navigate in real life. Our analysis of participant storytelling was sensitive also to the positioning of self, relationships and biopolitical citizenship (Squire 2013b) and, further, how such narrative can perform pandemic engagements, too.

In what follows we draw out three key lessons for public engagement with pandemic threats: persuasion narrative and its implications; how individuals addressed themselves to biopolitical citizenship in light of the 2009 pandemic, and; biopolitical metaphors—contagion and immunity—and their association with embodied individualism. We also consider a more general question of what our research suggests for the turn to narrative in public health with reference to the global nature of pandemics.

Knowing, Persuasion and Post-Trust Storytelling

Unlike states of illness, which depend on determinate biomedical diagnosis and the related transformation of identity and relationality, pandemic experience was most often indeterminate due to the infrequency with which influenza infection is diagnosed in a laboratory and the great variation in influenza symptoms between people, between influenza outbreaks, and even over the course of a particular influenza pandemic. In addition, the 2009 pandemic was mild for most people and many may have been infected without knowing. These qualities of influenza meant that experience of the pandemic in 2009 was highly reliant on television, print and online news, public health communications including websites, and notices in public buildings and public transport. The 2009 pandemic was therefore the apotheosis of a biocommunicable global health crisis (Briggs and Nichter 2009) and presented itself as an ideal case for exploring the nexus of narrative, publics, and the expert messaging of public health communications (Seale 2002).

An important feature of the 2009 pandemic as a biocommunicable health crisis was the discrepancy between what individuals said was media hype and the actual content of news media texts. As we noted in chapter 7, it is likely that media consumers in the United Kingdom, Australia, and elsewhere noticed that the H1N1 pandemic was a novel news story and that it was reported with great frequency over a short period of time. Another reason, however, for the attribution of hype to the news media and related skepticism was the generalized pandemic narrative itself. News media stories relied on and supported the pandemic narrative—the emergence, peak, and subsidence of public health emergency—by signaling alert in the first days of the pandemic's announcement and then sustaining the implied chance of catastrophe by simply repeating the message that the pandemic was in progress. News stories on the H1N1 pandemic were peopled with characters, most commonly the figure of the public health expert, who was reported to provide facts and figures regarding the pandemic. News media reliance on facts and figures and the expert voice of public health systems, then, was not simply a means of signifying and explaining the pandemic; it kept the pandemic alive by revealing the statistical and biomedical materialities of the virus's spread and effects. This aspect of news media deliberations on pandemic influenza is axiomatic to the force with which pandemic narrative asserts itself. The pandemic narrative implies the possibility of an emergent event even in the context of a subsiding pandemic, which always has within it the chance of resurgence. The content of the news stories, therefore, was less important than the overall shape of news media and their entanglements with pandemic experience in the media rich social worlds of the people in our interviews and focus groups (Kember and Zylinska 2015).

It is likely, too, that publics read or at least observed the news in the context of pandemic narratives circulating in popular culture, as Wald has suggested (2008), and were influenced by communications on previous health alerts (Ungar 2008). Our and other research participants seemed to have been skeptical by default, marking the high degree of familiarity and possible weariness with which they consumed the pandemic message (Joffe 2011). This idea of skeptical-as-usual publics is an important insight for public health. Reliance on facts and the voice of experts in news stories does not erase what has come before and, in particular, pandemic storytelling and the temporalized materiality of news storytelling. In this light, narrative public health is woven into the repetition of storytelling in English-language pandemic culture, at least, a feature of its existence with which it needs to contend to shape effective public engagement for the future.

Acceptance of the threat entailed in pandemic influenza was figured through what we have termed persuasion narrative, reversing the extant idea of narrative persuasion. The emergence of the pandemic in 2009 was spoken of as a gradual, largely media-dependent, awareness of the pandemic threat, articulated with the complexities of biographical and biomedical situation. News media narrative practices were important as they provided the means by which people reflected on the pandemic and its nuances and, where relevant, took on "at risk" identities and related action on their health situation. The example of Sarah, first introduced in chapter 2, who asked in her account, "Is it going to be real?," marked the invitation to pandemic citizenship implied in the alert message. Acceptance of this invitation was narrated as a graduated interpellation of risk subjectivity that left room for doubt but that also did not necessarily reject the public health message or foreclose action on the pandemic's risks. This way of talking about the pandemic sustained narrator identities as thoughtful and self-aware, creating scope for skepticism but also reasoned endorsement of public health advice on what members of the general public could do to avoid and manage influenza infection. This activation of persuasion narrative was particularly important for those who, like Sarah, came to learn that they may have been more "at risk" than others.

Our research participants took this skillful interpretation into their readings of the "Be alert, not alarmed" messaging that pervaded public health communications in 2009. Experts and government authorities appealed to publics to manage their affective response to the pandemic so that they did not overreact and therefore disrupt good governance, but also so that they did not lapse into complacency. This delicately balanced, Goldilocks message (Briggs and Nichter 2009), marked the construction of publics poised in useful readiness to act in case of serious public health emergency, or to threat more generally. As we indicated, this "Be alert, not alarmed" message is pervasive in global public health alerts, for example, in connection with Zika virus in 2016, and has a genealogy in previous biopolitical epochs where classed and gendered stoicism (Honigsbaum 2013), Cold War anxieties, and neoliberal flexibilization (Martin 1994) have been associated with responses to other pandemics and microbial threats. The provision of facts and figures in a news story or advice in campaign materials, then, does not simply transmit knowledge; it inscribes and circulates biopolitical assumptions of the relationships people have with expert knowledge. These different formulations of the ideal risk subject reveal how communication on a pandemic's dimensions, severity, and risks is also constitutive of the ideal citizenship of public life and, by implication, failed, unruly citizens. Media consumers potentially absorb the knowledge and advice provided but are also invited to choose between modes of citizenship.

Public trust in the expert knowledge systems and communications of public health are implicated in these narrative practices. The "Be alert, not alarmed" message is the frame for the circulation of facts and figures and reassuring messages from authorities that the emergency is in hand. A keynote of our analysis, however, was the critical awareness of this messaging in our interviews and focus groups. Communications on pandemic threats are hyperreflexive in the sense that publics and experts alike are aware of how what is said has ramifications for how expert knowledge is interpreted and applied. As we explored in chapter 8, however, the 2009 pandemic event, because it turned out to be milder than first thought, introduced the problem of "crying wolf" and related implications for the trustworthiness of pandemic messages. The deeply moralizing folktale of the untrustworthy shepherd boy was a way of narrating imperiled trust, as indicated in our interviews and focus groups. Hallin's and Brigg's idea of premediatization (2015) helped us to reflect on the thoroughly reflexive way in which media, communications, and pandemic narratives were organized to achieve biopolitical effects, and also that our participants were aware of this situation. In this view, the stories they told us of reading the "Be alert, not alarmed" message helped them to perform reflexive biopolitical citizenship, another way in which insights from narrative public health can be put to productive use.

Narrative Positioning and Pandemic Identities

Experience narrative on the 2009 pandemic influenza event was, as we have seen, complexly articulated with biography, personal biomedical circumstances, and social setting. Publics are convened under the sign of pandemic risk in ways that are both universal and particular: pandemic influenza is a risk that all may face, making it a problem of collective action for which identity does not matter and therefore complicating notions of biological citizenship that are held to be the basis for action on health problems (Rose and Novas 2005). But pandemic risk is also deeply individual, because preexisting health conditions and personal circumstances such as coincident pregnancy accentuate risk. This mixture of the universal and the particular divides individuals (Stephenson et al. 2014), as we have noted, in sometimes unhelpful ways and reveals some problems to do with public messaging. Our analysis therefore focused on the illumination of how people experienced and enacted being "at risk," or not. We also considered how they positioned themselves and others in their stories to reveal the significance of age, gender, and preexisting biomedical identities, but in ways that recognized the intersectional qualities of these experiences (Hankivsky 2012).

Unless faced with a preexisting health condition and or pregnancy, younger people in our research positioned themselves as unlikely to succumb to pandemic influenza. In contrast, older people made references to their lifetime experiences with other infectious diseases, including the introduction of polio vaccination. These situated, but strongly generational and temporalized engagements with pandemic influenza signaled the significance of the history of pandemics, the transformation of medicine, and expectations for health. To some extent pandemic communications have sought to address age and generation. For example, the CDC's use of zombie narrative to promote pandemic preparedness (Nasiruddin et al. 2013) has been justified in terms of offering greater appeal to young people than more traditional forms of health education. The younger people we spoke with readily spoke of influenza as a disease of the older and the vulnerable in ways that reinforced their own sense of themselves as having inherited a world where infectious diseases are less problematic for them. It seems to us, therefore, that zombie preparedness, for example, may not sufficiently address the historical and generational organization of responses to pandemic threat. Indeed, it may reinforce the idea that pandemic threat is distant for younger people who have no other health problems or who are not pregnant.

Gender also appeared to divide the enactment of expert advice on pandemic threat. The general pandemic message asks all to take action, but it is plain from our research that this generic message is mediated by gendered understandings of healthcare and responses to infectious diseases. The intensification of expectations on pregnant mothers in a time of pandemic was perhaps the clearest example, but the feminization of action on pandemic influenza was seen in other ways, including in relation to the labor of women to care for children and male partners and in the somewhat ambiguous metaphor of "man flu." Public responses to pandemics indicate that communications, styled as they are to address all as equal citizens, nevertheless mobilize the gendered ordering of health care. When a public health authority advises the general public to take action, then, the same message is read differently depending on one's gendered standpoint on healthcare and one's responsibilities to others. The feminization of the labor of action on pandemics is a likely effect that can go unchallenged.

People with preexisting health conditions also divided themselves from the "not at risk," but in ways that were particular to their situation. Pregnant women, as noted, found themselves at the intersection of gendered expectations of healthcare and their responsibilities as mothers to be, or new mothers. People with HIV, in contrast, spoke of H1N1 in terms of how it might have affected their HIV treatments or, as Heather (chapter 6) did, as relatively inconsequential in light of the threats to life faced by asylum seekers living with HIV and the more general effect of the HIV pandemic in Africa. People with respiratory illness were different again, and it seemed to us came close to a collective biological citizenship because their conditions were so directly implicated by the symptoms and risks of influenza. A key feature of these accounts was visibility and disclosure and a related biopolitical problem of being "at risk" and accepting that and how many others did not understand that they were potentially "a risk" to those with vulnerabilities. Indeed, the public communications on pandemic influenza were seen to be ambiguous in this sense, since they led some to think that their own vulnerability was trivialized and/or that "a risk" subjects were given reassurance, when their own status of being "at risk" continued.

The positioning that people take in their narratives and related intersectionalities to do with age, generation, gender, and health status are nuanced insights that can inform public health communications and/or help explain why they are effective for some individuals and groups but not others. Our analysis indicates, therefore, some of the benefits of taking an approach to public health communications that exploits the theory of subjective life developed by narrative analysts (Phoenix 2013, Squire 2013a).

Metaphor, Microbial Life and Immunopolitics

Pandemic narratives are placeholders for rich metaphors of life under threat. The metaphorical properties of contagion and immunity give pandemic narratives biopolitical resonance, connecting as they do: political imperatives to do with the production of life; the self defined and protected against the other; the *milieu interieur* scene for commune with microbial invaders and friends; the tensions implied in proximity and distance; and the coconstruction of narrative and knowledge. These resonances help explain why pandemic narratives have such carriage in public life, supplying ways of denoting and connoting collective and individual matters of life and death. These metaphors inform media texts, from public health advice, through literary and journalistic history, curated first-person narratives of pandemic experience, pulp fiction, zombie culture, and, as we have seen, to edutaining hybrids of public health interventions with popular culture. It is vital to be able to take a position on the biopolitical effects of these uses of pandemic metaphors. To fail to do so may contribute, as Wald has suggested, to blindness to unjust habits of thought and their effects (2008). A critical narrative public health is therefore crucial for enlarging options for action on pandemic matters and beyond.

Contagion metaphors help to exercise imaginaries of touch, networks, space, transmission, and social worlds and, in particular, the circulation of dangers, including ideas and infections. They supply the means of linking society, politics, and scientific knowledge about microbial threats. A key theme in our analysis was however the social distance ripple of the contagion metaphor. In this regard, research participants understood pandemic threats like influenza to travel across spaces that were both delimited and networked, giving ideas of social isolation used in public health a profoundly troublesome, improbable quality.

We also noted how narrative can be organized in ways that exact social distance in the sense of alienated audiences. For example, Rebecca, first introduced in chapter 3, referred to the named and unnamed expert "they" who feature in pandemic narrative. This reference to "they" was a recurring theme of our interviews and focus groups and marked another important feature of narrative on pandemics to do with its key actors and, through them and more abstractly, forms of agency. "They" are the experts who produce and disseminate knowledge of pandemics. Sometimes these experts are individuals named in news media such as chief health officers and senior government officials, but at other times "they" is a generalized expert source, an anonymous representative of science and its knowledge systems. This reference to the expert "they" signals how knowledge on pandemics is personified and attributed to human agency, be it the general "they" of personal experience narrative or the *dramatis personae* of news and popular culture pandemic narratives. This practice of narration also has the effect of inscribing relationality; of the relation between the narrator as layperson and the expert "they" who are in some ways distant and unknown, but nevertheless figure in reflections on how one should respond to a pandemic influenza threat. This relationality figures expertise as outside the self and therefore reinforces the dependence of individuals on the expert knowledge systems that are largely outside their control (Giddens 1990). This way of narrating influenza risk codifies the engagements of publics with the expert knowledge systems of public health and of contemporary life more generally.

The social distance between experts—"they"—and publics produced in pandemic communications and elsewhere may be inescapable. Much has been made of the importance of dialogue between public health and its publics for the purposes of more effective communications and to ward off the problem of mistrust. But how actually can dialogical communications happen, particularly in the early days of a global health threat, when news and other media are pivotal to the social response? More importantly, how has it come to be that public health, via its knowledge and communications practices, is distanciated from the publics it serves? Are there other ways of shaping public health that do not lead to the alienation of publics and experts? User-driven digital media may provide some methods for dialogical public—expert engagement and, as noted previously, references to "listening" to publics via digital media are being incorporated into pandemic preparedness policy documents (Australian Department of Health 2014, page 63). Knowledge of how best to employ participatory media in health, however, is only beginning to emerge (Wathen, Wyatt, and Harris 2008), as is inquiry on the narrative practices that digital media make possible (Georgakopolou 2014). Our narrative approach reveals the limits that pertain to the aspiration for dialogue, casting doubt on the idea that it is a communicative panacea. In addition, uncritical exploitation of concepts like narrative persuasion may help to emphasize social distance between those who formulate public health advice and those who receive it. Overcoming such social distance is something we have begun to explore in this book and it is an aspiration that connects up with "lay epidemiology" (Lovatt et al. 2015) and "counter public health" (Race 2009), concepts that seek to build public health approaches based on the views and lives of those most affected by ill-health. Similarly, edutainment in health and science communications tries to engage audiences, but as we have suggested, narrative distanciation may also circulate in these efforts.

Our analysis also explored the ways in which the uncertainties and strictly unavoidable qualities of influenza forced our research participants to reflect on their embodied resilience to infection and to articulate notions of personal immunity styled in the mode of acquisitive and individualized consumerism. Time and again in our focus groups and interviews, individuals endorsed ideas of hygiene and avoidance of the influenza virus, but because of the tensions of delimited and networked space noted above, all recognized that infection was likely. On the basis of this reasoning, participants spoke of their immunity, though not strictly in scientific terms. Immunity talk was akin to a mixture of scientific ideas of immunity and ideas of fortifying embodied resilience through self-care combined with the acquisition of consumer products. Significantly the idea that one's immune system was educable meant that traffic with microbial life was needed in order for the body to learn how to defend itself. This immunopolitics gave emphasis to the choices and conduct of the individual in the face of a microbial threat—such as pandemic influenza—over which they had limited control. Remarkably, then, the global effort to respond to a public health emergency of international concern in 2009 was translated into a focus of individuals on the interiors of their bodies and presumably unavoidable infection. The survival of individuals thrown back onto personal resources was the key note theme of this immunopolitical response. A related turn in this immunopolitics was the relative absence of ideas of being "a risk" to others and therefore of talk on, for example, herd immunity and vaccination to protect those seen to be more "at risk."

Strongly individualized and embodied immunopolitics have implications for the publics of public health. In the case of the 2009 pandemic, for example, did the public really matter in the sense of collective agency? What seemed to matter as a general public message was suspended agency or a conserved docility in the sense of readiness to act in case of a more serious turn in the pandemic's progress, that is, "be alert." This conception of the public in general of course made life difficult for those who were also, paradoxically, called up to take action because they were pregnant or otherwise "at risk." As we have seen, the gradual dawning of being "at risk" required considerable reflection on expert advice in media texts and was somewhat isolating. In addition, public health communications on pandemic threat appear to connect not with any collective sense of plight and peril, but with individuals in charge of themselves and (mostly for women it seemed) those for whom they provided care such as children and partners. These emphases in immunopolitical citizenship imply the erasure of public health publics. Pandemic alerts, therefore, may promote a way of life within which publics as an immunopolitical problem no longer matter. Charles McCoy (2016) has argued that the history of public health in the United Kingdom can be traced into knowledge generated by Edwin Chadwick and others in regard to the effects of poverty on health in the rapidly urbanizing cities of the industrial revolution. Contemporary immunopolitics however, looks to the embodied individual and *milieu interieur* to construct a very different notion of public health and its publics. This transition from public health concerned with the collective plight of those who suffer in economic systems to late modern corporeal individualism is not the same as the new public health (Petersen and Lupton 1996), which focuses on self-surveillance. This individualism also runs counter to public health approaches that emphasize mathematical modeling and therefore population-level management of health outcomes, as, for example, in HIV and the use of effective antiviral treatments to prevent new infections (Patton 2011). In immunopolitically organized public health, the individual is turned in on their embodied interiorities as a matter of surviving health threats for which they, medically and otherwise, are not able to take action.

These critiques have salience for new iterations of pandemic preparedness policy, developed in light of the 2009 swine flu pandemic, which appear to give emphasis to critical engagement on the part of members of the general public. The WHO has recommended that public health systems throughout the world "develop effective strategies to inform, educate and communicate with individuals and families to improve their ability to take appropriate actions before, during and after a pandemic" (2013, page 28). In the United Kingdom, the *Scientific Summary of Pandemic Influenza and Its Mitigation* says that, along with the action of the public health system, public health agencies should conduct "effective communication to the public, including skills training, to promote habits of stringent respiratory etiquette and hand hygiene, particularly amongst children" (Department of Health 2011, page 8). The 2014 UK *Pandemic Influenza Response Plan* (Public Health England 2014) features communications strategies at each step in the response, involving the provision of expert advice to professionals and members of the general population, monitoring of news media, press releases, and the use of social media such as Facebook and Twitter. The 2014 version of the *Australian Health Management Plan for Pandemic Influenza* says that "by giving the public up to date, consistent and accurate information about the status of the disease overseas and in Australia they can participate in managing the pandemic by taking steps to reduce the risk to themselves and their families" (Australian Department of Health 2014, page 12). The 2014 Australian plan depicted communications in this way:

> Communications measures should be commenced in order to mobilize responders and health services, and prepare the public for the impact of the disease, how it will be managed and how they can contribute to the response. Targeting of communication measures to vulnerable groups should be considered (Australian Department of Health 2014, page 45).

Later in the document, communications were depicted as methods to "engage, empower and build confidence in the community" (Australian

Department of Health 2014, page 49). Communications, then, are seen as vital to any effective response and have a political tone suggestive of the building of trust and therefore the production of compliant publics. It remains to be seen, however, whether these aspirational statements on the value of public engagement will be translated into effective action, particularly as they gloss over, as did previous policy framings, the underlying emphasis on personal immunity.

Toward Narrative Public Health

Narrative public health, however, need not only reinforce immunopolitical atomization. It can also look beyond the encouragement of individuals to take action, that is, persuading them through folktales of the microbial fates of heroes, victims, and villains and teaching, therefore, of character, cause and effect, and culpability. Narrative public health can also address itself to collective aspects of health problems by supplying an arena for critical reflection and productive action. As Paul Ricoeur suggested in a discussion of narrative and borrowing from Socrates, "an unexamined life is not worth living" (1991, page 20). By this he meant that narrative has its effects in its readings and that, by implication, life is experienced through its examination (Squire 2005, Wood 1991). These perspectives imply that narrative public health is useful, not to simply mediate knowledge and advice and persuade, but to assist with reflection on, for example, the individual and collective forms that immunopolitical life can take, as did many of the people in our interviews and focus groups.

This emphasis on critical reflection might be a vital role for narrative public health given that the center of gravity for the production of pandemic culture is not necessarily within the grasp of health communication professionals. For example, Nicole's Story, which we discussed in a previous chapter, is sophisticated YouTube marketing with production values that emulate cinema, qualities that may not be easy to reproduce in shrinking public health budgets. Edutainment for science and health hybridizes expert knowledge with popular culture, but printed, television, and online news media, as we have seen, appear to be important for coding and circulating the pandemic message, particularly in the early phases of a global health emergency. These perspectives imply that a fruitful role for narrative public health may not be found in competing with extensively resourced public pandemic culture but rather in offering audiences critical tools for navigating and decoding pandemic storytelling.

The turn to narrative in public health has salience, too, for global health. Our book has been tied to empirical material from the United Kingdom and Australia, but we have made reference to the globalizing qualities of influenza pandemics and examples such as HIV, Zika, and Ebola, all of which are revealed to affect the Global South and their transnational networks with the Global North. Our interviewees, too, in their reflections on pandemic influenza, spoke of news stories that depicted the infection emerging in other parts of the world, and some appeared to understand the 2009 pandemic as, simultaneously, personally relevant and global. These perspectives imply that the stories of infections that circulate in public and private life are imbued with the transnational connections of people, nonhuman animals, and other life. Central to our analysis were the key metaphors of contagion and immunity that helped to explain how people engaged with an emerging pandemic. For our interviewees, the complexities of geographic and social distance were figured around the impossibility of isolation and not actually resolved combinations of self-other and network immunities. The pandemic narrative, then, is already one of global networks and implications for life. An important dimension of narrative public health, then, is understanding how the pandemic narrative is deployed and reworked across transnational networks and in relation to the biological and social particularities of different infectious diseases.

The global network view also makes the emerging infectious diseases narrative appear somewhat northern-centric, since in the Global South, HIV, Zika, Ebola, and other infections are chronic and spreading or emerge recurrently. It would be unfortunate, then, if the Global North focused on preparedness while the Global South contended with the actualities of chronic and recurrent infectious diseases in ways that furthered the separation of the material and symbolic resources of North and South. Preparedness may be relevant for pandemic influenza and be otherwise a valuable policy tool, but global health needs to also look to present, in vivo capacities and initiatives for chronic and recurrent infections. Narrative public health, by implication, could serve different ways of telling the infectious diseases story that sponsor productive action for all in a networked world.

We started this book with reflections on the significance of narrative as a way of knowing and acting in a time of pandemic, as a tool of public health in its efforts to mitigate threats to life. There are all manner of ways in which pandemic narratives—across genres, media technologies, and public and private life—give meaning and help to organize the social response to a pandemic that evolves in an unpredictable manner. How else can we engage with an impending, uncertain, unseen threat if not through narrative imagination (Andrews 2014)? Narrative speculation on pandemic futures is also how we imagine futures in general, how they can be secured, and how human agency can be cultivated for survival. Our deliberation on what the 2009 pandemic might imply for narrative public health is no doubt only a starting point for further inquiry, reflection, and action. How to live with microbial life is an age-old problem, cast as new in narratives on life-threatening pandemics, relentlessly emerging infectious diseases, and the superbugs apocalypse, as the media has dubbed it. As our research participants suggested, living in productive ways with microbial life are stories that can also be told and that may be vital methods for creating livable futures.

References

Andrews, M. 2014. *Narrative imagination and everyday life, explorations in narrative psychology*. New York: Oxford University Press.
Australian Department of Health. 2014. *Australian health management plan for pandemic influenza*. Canberra: Commonwealth of Australia.
Belling, C. 2009. "Overwhelming the medium: Fiction and the trauma of pandemic influenza in 1918." *Literature & Medicine* 28 (1):55–81.
Briggs, C, and M Nichter. 2009. "Biocommunicability and the biopolitics of pandemic threats." *Medical Anthropology* 28 (3):189–198.
Department of Health. 2011. *Scientific summary of pandemic influenza and its mitigation*. London: Pandemic Influenza Preparedness Team.
Georgakopolou, A. 2014. "Small stories transposition and social media: A microperspective on the 'Greek crisis.'" *Discourse & Society* 25 (4):519–539.
Giddens, A. 1990. *The consequences of modernity*. Cambridge: Polity.
Hallin, Daniel C, and Charles L Briggs. 2015. "Transcending the medical/media opposition in research on news coverage of health and medicine." *Media, Culture & Society* 37 (1):85–100. doi: 10.1177/0163443714549090.
Hankivsky, O. 2012. "Women's health, men's health, and gender and health: Implications of intersectionality." *Social Science & Medicine* 74 (11):1712–1720.
Hilton, S, and K Hunt. 2011. "UK newspapers' representation of the 2009–10 outbreak of swine flu: One health scare not over-hyped by the media?" *Journal of Epidemiology and Community Health* 65:941–946.
Honigsbaum, M. 2013. "Regulating the 1918–19 pandemic: Flu, STOICISM and the Northcliffe Press." *Medical History* 57 (2):165–185. doi: http://dx.doi.org/10.1017/mdh.2012.101.
Joffe, H. 2011. "Public apprehension of emerging infectious diseases: Are changes afoot?" *Public Understanding of Science* 20 (4):446–460.

Kember, S, and J Zylinska. 2015. *Life after new media: Mediation as a vital process*. Cambridge, MA: MIT Press.

Lovatt, M, D Eadie, P Meier, J Li, L Bauld, G Hastings, and J Holmes. 2015. "Lay epidemiology and the interpretation of low-risk drinking guidelines by adults in the United Kingdom." *Addiction* 110:1912–1919.

Martin, E. 1994. *Flexible bodies: Tracking immunity in American culture from the days of polio to the age of AIDS*. Boston: Beacon Press.

McCoy, C. 2016. "SARS, pandemic influenza and Ebola: The disease control styles of Britain and the United States." *Social Theory & Health* 14 (1):1–17.

Nasiruddin, M, M Halabi, A Dao, K Chen, and B Brown. 2013. "Zombies—A pop culture resource for public health awareness." *Emerging Infectious Diseases* 19:809+.

Patton, C. 2011. "Rights language and HIV treatment: Universal care or population control?" *Rhetoric Society Quarterly* 41 (3):250–266.

Petersen, A, and D Lupton. 1996. *The new public health: Health and self in the age of risk*. St Leonards, NSW: Allen & Unwin.

Petersen, A, M Davis, S Fraser, and J Lindsay. 2010. "Healthy living and citizenship: An overview." *Critical Public Health* 20 (4):391–400.

Phoenix, A. 2013. "Analysing narrative contexts." In *Doing narrative research, second edition*, edited by M Andrews, C Squire, and M Tamboukou, 72–87. London: Sage.

Public Health England. 2014. *Pandemic influenza response plan, 2014*. London: Public Health England.

Race, K. 2009. *Pleasure consuming medicine: The queer politics of drugs*. Durham: Duke University Press.

Ricoeur, P. 1991. "Life in quest of narrative." In *On Paul Ricoeur: Narrative and interpretation*, edited by D Wood, 20–22. London: Routledge.

Rose, N, and C Novas. 2005. "Biological citizenship." In *Global assemblages: Technology, politics, and ethics as anthropological problems*, edited by A Ong and S Collier, 439–463. Malden, MA: Blackwell.

Seale, C. 2002. *Media and health*. London: Sage.

Squire, C. 2005. "Reading narratives." In "Contemporary social theory," special issue, edited by E. Burman and S. Frosh. *Group Analysis* 38 (1):91–107.

Squire, C. 2013a. "From experience-centred to socioculturally-oriented approaches to narrative." In *Doing narrative research, second edition*, edited by M Andrews, C Squire, and M Tamboukou, 47–71. London: Sage.

Squire, C. 2013b. *Living with HIV and ARVs: Three letter lives*. Houndmills: Palgrave Macmillan.

Squire, C, M Davis, C Esin, M Andrews, B Harrison, L Hyden, and M Hyden. 2014. *What is narrative research?* London: Bloomsbury Academic.

Stephenson, N, M Davis, P Flowers, E Waller, and C MacGregor. 2014. "Mobilising 'vulnerability' in the public health response to pandemic influenza." *Social Science & Medicine* 102:10–17.

Ungar, Sheldon. 2008. "Global bird flu communication: Hot crisis and media reassurance." *Science Communication* 29 (4):472–497.

Wald, P. 2008. *Contagious: Cultures, carriers, and the outbreak narrative*. Durham: Duke University Press.

Wathen, N, S Wyatt, and R Harris, eds. 2008. *Mediating health information: The go-betweens in a changing socio-technical landscape*. Houndmills: Palgrave Macmillan.

Wood, D. 1991. "Introduction: Interpreting narrative." In *On Paul Ricouer: Narrative and interpretation*, edited by D Wood, 1–19. London: Routledge.

World Health Organization. 2013. *Pandemic Influenza Risk Management: WHO Interim Guidance*. Geneva: World Health Organization.

APPENDIX 1

Participants Who Appear in the Text, with References to Relevant Chapters

Pseudonym	Location	Age	Group	Chapters
Alex	Sydney	30s	Lung disease	5
Angela	Melbourne	30s	Pregnant in 2009	4
Anne and Gary	Melbourne	Anne: 60s Gary: 70s	Anne: No disclosed health problems Gary: Chronic illness	5
Archie	Sydney	60s	Lung disease	5
Bobby	Glasgow	40s	HIV positive	3
Brigitte	Melbourne	40s	No disclosed health problems	4, 6
Cameron	Glasgow	40s	No disclosed health problems	1, 8
Chris	Melbourne	20s	No disclosed health problems	6
Cindy	Sydney	20s	Lung disease	4, 6, 8
Claire	Glasgow	30s	Pregnant in 2009	4, 6, 7, 8
Dave	Glasgow	60s	No disclosed health problems	3
Deb	Melbourne	30s	New baby in 2009	3, 4
Diane	Melbourne	50s	Severe illness on 2009	4
Gill	Melbourne	30s	Pregnant in 2009	3, 4, 6
Gordon	Melbourne	60s	Lung disease	4, 5
Jenny and Simon	Melbourne	Jenny: 60s Simon: 50s	Jenny: Lung disease Simon: Chronic illness	4
Katrina	Melbourne	70s	Older group	6
Lara	Sydney	30s	Lung disease	3
Linda	Sydney	30s	Pregnant in 2009	8
Liz and Peter	Melbourne	50s	No disclosed health problems	7, 8
Lizzy	Glasgow	20s	No disclosed health problems	6
Lola	Melbourne	60s	No disclosed health problems	5
Margaret	Melbourne	70s	Older group	6
Marie	Sydney	20s	No disclosed health problems	6, 8
Marilyn	Melbourne	30s	Pregnant in 2009	6, 8
Marlene	Sydney	30s	Lung disease	3, 6

Pseudonym	Location	Age	Group	Chapters
Mary	Glasgow	30s	Pregnant in 2009	3, 4, 8
Matrix	Glasgow	50s	HIV positive	5, 6
Maude	Glasgow	30s	Pregnant in 2009	4, 5
Mitzi	Sydney	30s	Lung disease	5, 6
Nicole	Sydney	20s	Lung disease	4
Pippa	Sydney	30s	Lung disease	6
Rebecca	Glasgow	30s	Pregnant in 2009	3, 6, 8
Rob	Melbourne	40s	HIV positive	5
Roslyn	Melbourne	60s	No disclosed health problems	4, 5, 6
Sarah	Glasgow	30s	Pregnant in 2009	2, 4, 6, 7
Vaughn	Sydney	20s	No disclosed health problems	7, 8
Vincent	Sydney	40s	No disclosed health problems	3, 6
Xavier	Sydney	30s	No disclosed health problems	4
Focus group: Arthur	Melbourne	60s and 70s	Lung disease	6
Focus group: Beatrice, Hannah, Pauline, Bob, Suzanne	Sydney	50s and 60s	Lung disease	8
Focus group: Heather, Beth	Glasgow	30s, 40s, 50s	HIV positive	6
Focus group: Lachlan and Jason	Melbourne	20s	No disclosed health problems	7
Focus group: Natalie	Melbourne	20s	No disclosed health problems	6
Focus group: Rachel, Sabrina, Lisa, Abbie	Sydney	40s and 50s	No disclosed health problems	5
Focus group: Sally, Melanie, Josh, Oscar	Melbourne	20s	No disclosed health problems	5
Focus group: Simon, Dean	Glasgow	30s, 40s, 50s	HIV positive	6

Index

Tables, figures and boxes are indicated by *t*, *f* and *b* following the page number
For the benefit of digital users, indexed terms that span two pages (e.g., 52–53) may, on occasion, appear on only one of those pages.

activism, alliances in, 27
advertisements, in 2009 pandemic, 51–52
age
   and conceptualizations of invulnerability, 123–27
   and configurations of vulnerability, 119–22
   polio, attitudes toward, 125–27
   and visible vulnerability, 138
Alibek, K., *Biohazard,* 22–23
alienation, social distancing and, 75–76
antiviral treatment, 72–73
anxiety, titrating public, 59–64
Australia
   approach to research in, 11
   costs of addressing 2009 pandemic, 166–67
   critical awareness of preparedness messaging, 54–55, 58–59
   framing of news media accounts in, 151–52
   HIV public education campaigns in, 26–27
   influenza pandemic of 2009, news media stories, 148–50, 149*t*
   influenza pandemic of 2009 in, 9–10
   James Bishop, chief medical officer of, 46–47
   mortality rates in 2009 influenza pandemic, 164–65
   and mythical distance from pandemics, 80–85
   2009 pandemic, government review of response, 169
   policy configurations of vulnerability, 120–21
   preparedness citizenship in, 64–68
   preparedness planning, 33–35, 46–47
   public communications on 2009 pandemic, 49–50, 52–53
   public health communications in, 25–26
   school closings in, 72

biocommunicability, 30–31
Biohazard (Alibek & Handelman), 22–23
biomedicalization, of power, 31–32
biopower
   and metaphors of contagion *vs.* immunity, 36–37
   notion of, 30, 31–32
bioterrorism, government response to threat of, 28–29
Bishop, James, chief medical officer of Australia, 46–47
Bourdain, A., *Typhoid Mary: An Urban Historical,* 22–23
Briggs, Charles, biomedicalization of power, 31–32

Camus, Albert, *The Plague,* 23
Canada, mortality rates in 2009 pandemic, 164–65
Centers for Disease Control and Prevention (CDC)
   personal accounts of 1918 and 1957 influenza outbreaks, 22–23
   "zombie preparedness" program, 28
choice immunity, 106–16

chronic illness
  and conceptualizations of vulnerability, 134–37
  narrative positioning and, 193–94
  narratives of, 7–8
  and personal cultivation of immunity, 109–10
  and social distancing to avoid contagion, 89, 104–5, 106
  and visible vulnerability, 137–38, 139–41
Clinton, William Jefferson, 28–29
Cohen, Edward, culture of immunity, 99–100
collective immunity, 115–16
communication
  alertness *vs.* alarm in, 35–36, 46–48
  biocommunicability, 30–31
  contagion *vs.* immunity, metaphors of, 36–37
  direct-to-household, 177–78
  framing of, 147, 150–52
  hero *vs.* villain in, 36
  and narrative public health, 199–201
  and perceived false alarms, 170–78
  persuasion narrative, 156–60, 190–91
  premediatization of, 169
  preparedness messages, 198–99
  public trust in, 184, 191–92
  social and personal context for, 68–69
  strategies of, 146–47
  See also health communication; pandemic communication
communication, on 2009 pandemic, 48–53
  Australia, 49–50, 52–53
  critical awareness of, 53–59
  and preparedness citizenship, 64–69
  self-triage telephone services, 50–51
  television advertisements, 51–52
  titrating public panic, 59–64, 152–56
  United Kingdom, 48–49, 50–52
contagion, 72–76
  antiviral treatment in pandemics, 72–73
  biopolitical rationalities and, 73–74
  distancing from sources of, 76–80
  immunity as response to potential, 90–91
  metaphors of, 195
  mythical distances from, 80–85
  and narrative distanciation, 75–76
  and othering in pandemic narratives, 77
  and preparedness messages, 92
  psychosocial responses to, 17
  quarantine to avoid, 74
  social distancing, negotiable and partial, 85–93
  social distancing to avoid, 72–73, 76
  social distancing to avoid, 2009 influenza pandemic, 74–75
  vs. immunity in pandemic narratives, 36–37
Contagion (Soderbergh, 2011), 23
corporeality, of pandemic experience, 39–40
critical awareness, of preparedness messages, 53–59
"crying wolf," reference to folktale of, 171

Darabont, F., *The Walking Dead*, 23
Defoe, Daniel, *A Journal of the Plague Year*, 22–23
distanciation, and social distancing, 75–76
  in news media accounts of pandemics, 79–80
  pandemics, mythical distance from, 80–85
Donaldson, Liam, chief medical officer of United Kingdom, 46–47

E-Bug Detective Game, The (Farrell et al.), 28–29
economic differentiation
  in HIV pandemic, 26–27
  in influenza pandemic of 1918, 31–32
elderly populations, and influenza pandemic of 2009, 9–10
emergence of pandemics, discovering, 1
Epidemic That Never Was, The (Neustadt & Fineberg), 34–35, 167–68
Epstein, Steven, history of HIV science and treatment activism, 27
Europe, mortality rates in 2009 pandemic, 164–65

face masks, to avoid contagion, 74
Farmer, Paul, biomedicalizing power, 31–32
Farrell, D., *The E-Bug Detective Game,* 28–29
Fenn, E., *Pox Americana: The Great Smallpox Epidemic of 1775-82,* 22–23
Fineberg, Harvey, *The Epidemic That Never Was,* 34–35, 167–68
Flu: The Story of the Great Influenza Pandemic of 1918 and the Search for the Virus that Caused It (Kolata), 22–23
focus groups, and approach to research, 13–15
folktales, undercurrents in pandemic narratives, 35–37
Foucault, Michel
  on biopower, 30
  on security, 74
  security of the social, 100

gender
  and "man flu," 130–32
  and understandings of health care, 193
gender relations, and conceptualizations of invulnerability, 128–32
genetics research, activism and alliances in, 27
global health, and narrative public health, 200
globalization, and practicalities of social distancing, 75

Haiti, biomedicalization of power in, 31–32
Handelman, S., *Biohazard,* 22–23
Haraway, Donna, culture of immunity, 99–100
health communication
  alertness *vs.* alarm in, 35–36, 46–48
  biopolitical context of, 26, 30–31, 36–37
  contagion *vs.* immunity, metaphors of, 36–37
  direct-to-household, 177–78
  framing of, 147, 150–52
  hero *vs.* villain in, 36

historical, literary, and journalistic examples, 22–23
  narrative approaches to, 22–24, 25–28
  and narrative public health, 199–201
  and perceived false alarms, 170–78
  persuasion narrative, 156–60, 190–91
  popular culture and social media, 28
  premediatization of, 169
  preparedness messages, 198–99
  public trust in, 184, 191–92
  social and personal context for, 68–69
  strategies of, 146–47
health communication, on 2009 pandemic, 48–53
  Australia, 49–50, 52–53
  critical awareness of, 53–59
  and preparedness citizenship, 64–69
  self-triage telephone services, 50–51
  television advertisements, 51–52
  titrating public panic, 59–64, 152–56
  United Kingdom, 48–49, 50–52
hindsight, in narrative inquiry, 5
HIV pandemic
  advice on parenting in context of, 29–30
  and configurations of vulnerability, 120–22
  medicalized lives and, 134–36
  narrative positioning and, 193–94
  science and treatment activism, 27
  social and economic differentiation in, 26–27
  and visible vulnerability, 137–39
Hong Kong, 2003 SARS outbreak in, 74
Honigsbaum, M., immunity as consumer objective, 97–98

imagination, in narrative inquiry, 5
immunity, 96–98
  acquisition of, 110–15
  benefits of social interaction for, 106
  biomedical definition of, 99–100
  choice immunity, 106–16
  collective immunity, 115–16
  as consumer objective, 97–98
  culture of, 76–77
  "immune-boosting," 107–8
  immunity culture, 98
  interactive complexity of, 100

immunity (*cont.*)
   isolation and, 104–6
   as metaphor in pandemic
      narratives, 96–97
   news media messages on, 101
   origins of term, 99–100
   personal cultivation of, 106–16, 196–98
   personal experience narratives on,
      100–1, 102
   and preparedness messages, 103
   psychosocial perceptions of, 17
   resorting to, 99–103
   as response to potential
      contagion, 90–91
   vs. contagion in pandemic
      narratives, 36–37
immunopolitics
   of Global North, 98, 200
   and pandemic narratives, 196–98
infections, narrative inquiry on, 24
influenza, "man flu" and, 130–32
influenza outbreak, of 1976
   and public trust in preparedness
      messages, 167–68
   use in preparedness planning, 34–35
influenza outbreak of 1957, personal
      accounts of, 22–23
influenza pandemic, of 1918
   personal accounts of, 22–23
   political and historical context of, 26
   social and economic differentiation
      in, 31–32
   titrating public panic, 61
   use in preparedness planning, 33–34
influenza pandemic, of 2009, 8–11
   alertness *vs.* alarm in response to,
      35–36, 46–48
   critical awareness of public
      messaging, 53–59
   influencing individual behaviors
      during, 25–26
   mortality rates, 164–65
   news media stories on, 148–50, 148–50*t*
   particularities of, 9–10
   personal account, United
      Kingdom, 37–40
   preparedness citizenship, 64–69
   public trust afterward, 164–70

   as reflexive emergency, 9
   research, approach to, 11–16
   risk for pregnant women in, 132–33
   social distancing and, 76
   social response to, 2
   titrating public panic, 61, 152–56
   viruses, mutability and variation
      among, 10
   WHO surveillance of, 9
interviews, and approach to
      research, 13–15
invulnerability, conceptualizations
      of, 122–43
   contextualization of, 122–23
   gender relations and, 128–32
   invisibility of vulnerability, 137–43
   medicalized lives, 134–37
   pregnancy and, 132–34
   temporality and, 124–27
   vaccination and, 128–29
Ironstone-Catterall, Penelope, modulation
      of public anxiety, 59–60
isolation, and achieving immunity, 104–6

Journal of the Plague Year, A
   (Defoe), 22–23

Kolata, G., *Flu: The Story of the Great
   Influenza Pandemic of 1918 and
   the Search for the Virus that Caused
   It*, 22–23

Love Lines, parenting advice
   program, 29–30

Mantini-Briggs, Clara, biomedicalization
      of power, 31–32
"March of Dimes, The," 26
Martin, Emily, culture of immunity,
      76–77, 99–100
medicalized lives, and conceptualizations
      of vulnerability, 134–37
medicine
   narrative medicine, 24
   public trust in vaccination
      efforts, 178–84
metaphor, and pandemic
      narratives, 194–95

microbial life, and pandemic narratives, 194–99, 200–1
mortality rates, of 2009 influenza pandemic, 164–65
My Life with Flu, radio drama, 28–29
mythical distance, and emergence of pandemics, 80–85

narrative analysis, types of, 15
narrative approaches, advantages of, 28–29
narrative distanciation, and social distancing, 75–76
narrative inquiry, features of
  hindsight, 5
  imagination, 5
  narrative analysis, types of, 15
  temporality, coded, 5
narrative inquiry, on infections, 24
narrative medicine, 24
narrative persuasion, critiques of, 29–30
narrative positioning, 192–94
narrative public health, 17, 199–201
narratives
  absence of personal accounts, 2
  assistance in pandemics, 1
  biopolitical context of, 36–37
  of chronic illness, 7–8
  and corporeality of pandemic experience, 39–40
  folktale undercurrents in, 35–37
  forms of, 1–2
  and government response to threat of bioterrorism, 28–29
  in health communication, 25–28
  historical, literary, and journalistic examples, 22–23
  narrative analysis, types of, 15
  open-endedness of, 6–7
  personal account of 2009 influenza pandemic, United Kingdom, 37–40
  personal accounts of 1918 and 1957 influenza outbreaks, 22–23
  personal reality described in, 5–6
  psychosocial dimensions of, 6, 8
  and shaping of health and illness, 23–24
  speculation and prediction in, 32–35, 200–1

of "swine flu" pandemic, 4, 8–11
See also pandemic narratives
Neustadt, Richard, *The Epidemic That Never Was*, 34–35, 167–68
news media, accounts of pandemics, 32–33, 146–48
  distanciation and social distancing in, 79–80
  hyperbole in, 147–48, 150–51, 152–56
  immunity, messages on, 101
  influenza pandemic of 2009, 148–50, 148–49t, 150t
  and pandemic narratives, 189–90
  panic, titrating public, 152–56
  and personal realization of vulnerability, 38–39
  persuasion narrative, 156–60, 190–91
  public health communication, framing of, 147, 150–52
  public health communication, strategies of, 146–47
  and public trust in management of pandemics, 165, 191–92
  social and geographic distancing in, 91
  social distancing as reaction to, 82

Obama, Barrack H., response to "swine flu" pandemic, 35–36
open-endedness, of narrative, 6–7
Oshinsky, D., *Polio: An American Story*, 22–23
othering, in pandemic narratives, 31, 77, 84–85

pandemic communication
  alertness *vs.* alarm in, 35–36, 46–48
  biopolitical context of, 26, 30–31, 36–37
  challenges of, 17
  contagion *vs.* immunity, metaphors of, 36–37
  direct-to-household, 177–78
  engagement with, 3–4
  framing of, 147, 150–52
  hero *vs.* villain in, 36
  narrative and, 25–28
  narrative approaches to, 22–24
  and narrative public health, 199–201
  and perceived false alarms, 170–78

pandemic communication (*cont.*)
  popular culture and social media, 28
  premediatization of, 169
  preparedness messages, 198–99
  public reception of, 17
  public trust in, 184, 191–92
  social and personal context for, 68–69
  strategies of, 146–47
pandemic communication, on 2009 pandemic, 48–53
  Australia, 49–50, 52–53
  critical awareness of, 53–59
  and preparedness citizenship, 64–69
  self-triage telephone services, 50–51
  television advertisements, 51–52
  titrating public panic, 59–64, 152–56
  United Kingdom, 48–49, 50–52
pandemic culture, 98
pandemic experience
  corporeality of, 39–40
  intersection of history and biography, 120, 143
pandemic identities, 192–94
pandemic narratives
  absence of personal accounts, 2
  alertness *vs.* alarm in, 35–36, 46–48
  assistance from, 1
  assumptions and habits of thought in, 31
  and chronic illness, 7–8
  contagion *vs.* immunity, metaphors of, 36–37
  and corporeality of pandemic experience, 39–40
  distanciation in, 80
  engagements across public life, 188–89
  folktale undercurrents in, 35–37
  foretelling future in, 77
  forms of, 1–2
  gender, and understandings of health care, 193
  hero *vs.* villain in, 36
  immunity, metaphor of, 96–97
  immunity, personal cultivation of, 196–98
  metaphor and, 194–95
  narrative analysis, types of, 15
  and narrative positioning, 192–94
  and narrative public health, 199–201
  news media and, 189–90
  open-endedness of, 6–7
  othering in, 31, 77, 84–85
  and pandemic identities, 192–94
  personal account of 2009 influenza pandemic, United Kingdom, 37–40
  personal accounts of 1918 and 1957 influenza outbreaks, 22–23
  personal reality described in, 5–6
  and persuasion narrative, 190–91
  in popular culture, 23
  preparedness messages and, 198–99
  psychosocial dimensions of, 6, 8
  social distance and, 195–96
  speculation and prediction in, 32–35, 200–1
  of "swine flu" pandemic, 4, 8–11
  undercurrents and significance of, 16
pandemics
  discovering emergence of, 1
  mythical distance from, 80–85
  public trust in management of, 164–70, 173–74, 184, 191–92
  public trust in management of, and perceived false alarms, 170–78
  public trust in management of, vaccination efforts, 178–84
pandemics, speculation on future of, 32–35
  folktale undercurrents, 35–37, 171
  and narrative public health, 200–1
  preparedness planning, 33–35
  recollection of past pandemics, 33–35
panic, titrating public, 59–64, 105, 152–56
personal experience narratives
  absence of, 2
  on acquisition of immunity, 110–15
  age and invulnerability, 123–27
  on 1918 and 1957 influenza outbreaks, 22–23
  chronic illness and, 7–8
  and corporeality of pandemic experience, 39–40
  on enactment of social distance, 77–79, 80–92
  folktale undercurrents in, 35–37
  gender relations and invulnerability, 128–32

on "immune-boosting," 107–8
on immunity, 100–1, 102, 104–6
2009 influenza pandemic, United
    Kingdom, 37–40
introduction of, 2–8
"man flu," recollections of, 130–32
medicalized lives, 135–37
narrative analysis, types of, 15
news media accounts of
    pandemic, 153–54
open-endedness of, 6–7
and perceived false alarms, 171–78
on personal cultivation of
    immunity, 107–14
personal reality described in, 5–6
and persuasion narrative,
    157–59, 190–91
psychosocial dimensions of, 6, 8
and public trust in vaccination
    efforts, 178–84
of "swine flu" pandemic, 4, 8–11
on visible vulnerability, 138–39, 140–42
persuasion, critiques of narrative, 29–30
persuasion narrative
    and news media accounts,
        156–60, 190–91
    and pandemic narratives, 190–91
Plague, The (Camus), 23
polio
    age and attitudes toward, 125–27
    public education and marketing
        campaigns, 26
Polio: An American Story
    (Oshinsky), 22–23
popular culture
    pandemic narratives in, 23
    and public health communication, 28
power, biomedicalization of, 31–32
*Pox Americana: The Great Smallpox
    Epidemic of 1775-82* (Fenn), 22–23
"Precautionary Principle: Plan for the
    Worst, Hope for the Best, The"
    (WHO), 168–69
preexisting illness, and conceptualizations
    of vulnerability, 134–37
pregnancy
    and conceptualizations of
        vulnerability, 132–34

critical awareness of public
    messaging, 55–57
and influenza pandemic of 2009,
    9–10, 132–33
and pandemic narratives, 7–8
and personal account of 2009 influenza
    pandemic, 37–40
in policy configurations of
    vulnerability, 120–21
and public trust in vaccination
    efforts, 180–84
social distancing to avoid
    contagion, 85–89
and visible vulnerability, 138
preparedness messages
    and concept of immunity, 103
    contagion and, 92
    critical awareness of, 53–59
    and pandemic narratives, 198–99
    and perceived false alarms, 170–78
    and preparedness citizenship, 64–69
    public trust in, 164–70, 191–92
    social and personal context for, 68–69
preparedness planning, 33–35, 46–47
psychosocial dimensions, of narrative
    and approaches to research, 14–15
    opportunities to explore, 6
    personal experience and, 8
psychosocial responses, to contagion, 17
public health, collective dedication
    to, 26–27
public health approaches
    and influencing individual
        behaviors, 25–26
    in United Kingdom vs United
        States, 11–12
public health communication
    direct-to-household, 177–78
    framing of, 147, 150–52
    and narrative public health, 199–201
    and perceived false alarms, 170–78
    persuasion narrative, 156–60, 190–91
    popular culture and social media, 28
    premediatization of, 169
    preparedness messages, 198–99
    public trust in, 184, 191–92
    social and personal context for, 68–69
    strategies of, 146–47

public health communication, on 2009
    pandemic, 48–53
  Australia, 49–50, 52–53
  critical awareness of, 53–59
  and preparedness citizenship, 64–69
  self-triage telephone services, 50–51
  television advertisements, 51–52
  titrating public panic, 59–64, 152–56
  United Kingdom, 48–49, 50–52
public health institutions, educational
    campaigns, 28
public messaging, critical awareness of, 53–59
publics
  persuasion narrative and, 160, 190–91
  social and economic differentiation
    of, 26–27, 31–32
  trust in management of pandemics,
    164–70, 191–92

quarantine, and avoiding contagion, 74

Rabinow, Paul, science and treatment
    activism, 27
recollection, of past pandemics and
    events, 33–35
research, approach to, 11–16
  in Australia, 11
  focus groups, 13–15
  interviews, 13–15
  narrative analysis, types of, 15
  psychosocial dimensions of, 14–15
  in Scotland, 11–12
  volunteers, characteristics of, 12–13, 16
  volunteers, recruitment of, 12
research, articles resulting from, 14

schools, closings to avoid contagion, 72
Scotland, approach to research in, 11–12
Seale, Clive, narrative shaping of health
    and illness, 23–24
Security, Territory, Population
    (Foucault), 74
self-triage telephone services, in 2009
    pandemic, 50–51
severe acute respiratory syndrome (SARS),
    2003 outbreak, 74
social differentiation
  in HIV pandemic, 26–27
  in influenza pandemic of 1918, 31–32

social distancing, to avoid contagion, 72–73
  alienation and, 75–76
  in chronic illness, 89
  globalization and, 75
  negotiable and partial social
    distance, 85–93
  and pandemic narratives, 195–96
  practicalities of, 73
  in pregnancy, 85–89
  as reaction to news media, 82
  and sources of contagion, 76–80
  value of in 2009 influenza
    pandemic, 74–75
social interaction, benefits for
    immunity, 106
social media, and public health
    communication, 28
social response, to influenza pandemic of
    2009, 2
Soderbergh, S., *Contagion*, 23
Sontag, Susan, sources of contagion, 76–77
"Spanish Influenza," naming of, 26
stereotypes, in pandemic narratives, 31
"swine flu" pandemic, 8–11
  alertness *vs.* alarm in response to,
    35–36, 46–48
  particularities of, 9–10
  personal narrative of, 4
  as reflexive emergency, 9
  research, approach to, 11–16
  social response to, 2
  viruses, mutability and variation
    among, 10
  WHO surveillance of, 9

telephone services, in 2009
    pandemic, 50–51
television advertisements, in 2009
    pandemic, 51–52
temporality
  coded in narrative, 5
  and conceptualizations of
    invulnerability, 124–27
Toronto, Canada, 2003 quarantine for
    SARS, 74
Treichler, Paula, sources of
    contagion, 76–77
Typhoid Mary: An Urban Historical
    (Bourdain), 22–23

Ungar, Sheldon, news media and pandemics, 32–33
United Kingdom
 costs of addressing 2009 pandemic, 166–67
 critical awareness of preparedness messaging, 55–58
 framing of news media accounts in, 150–51
 HIV public education campaigns in, 26–27
 influenza pandemic of 2009, news media stories, 148–50, 149t
 influenza pandemic of 2009 in, 9–10
 Liam Donaldson, chief medical officer of, 46–47
 mortality rates in 2009 influenza pandemic, 164–65
 My Life with Flu, radio drama, 28–29
 personal account of 2009 influenza pandemic, 37–40
 policy configurations of vulnerability, 120–21
 preparedness planning, 33–35, 46–47
 public communications on 2009 pandemic, 48–49, 50–52
 public health approaches in, 11–12
 public health communications in, 25–26
 school closings in, 72
 titrating public panic, 62–64
United States, public health approaches in, 11–12

vaccination
 adverse reactions in influenza outbreak of 1976, 34–35
 age and attitudes toward, 123–27
 and conceptualizations of invulnerability, 128–29
 critical awareness of public messaging, 55–57
 gender relations and, 128–32
 narratively oriented communications on, 28–29
 participant history of, 13
 pregnancy and attitudes toward, 133–34
 and psychosocial perceptions of immunity, 17
 and public trust in management of pandemics, 165–66, 178–84
 as response to potential contagion, 90
Venezuela, biomedicalization of power in, 31–32
viruses, mutability and variation among, 10
volunteers
 characteristics of, 12–13
 recruitment for research, 12
vulnerabilities, 119–22
 contextualization of, 121–22
 gender relations and, 128–32
 invisibility of, 137–43
 invulnerability, contextualization of, 122–23
 medicalized lives, 134–37
 personal realization of, 38–39
 policy configurations of, 120–21
 pregnancy, 120–21, 132–34
 risks of revealing, 142–43
 temporality and, 124–27
 tiered approach to, 119–20
 workplace, visibility in, 141

Walking Dead, The (Darabont, 2010), 23
War of the Worlds (Wells), 23, 96–97
Wells, H. G., *War of the Worlds*, 23, 96–97
Wilbraham, Lindy, on narrative persuasion, 29–30
workplace, visible vulnerabilities in, 141
World Health Organization (WHO)
 and influenza mortality rates, 164–65
 and management of 2009 pandemic, 166–67, 168–69
 and surveillance of 2009 influenza pandemic, 9
 "The Precautionary Principle: Plan for the Worst, Hope for the Best," 168–69

young adults, and influenza pandemic of 2009, 9–10

Zika virus, biomedicalization of power and, 31–32

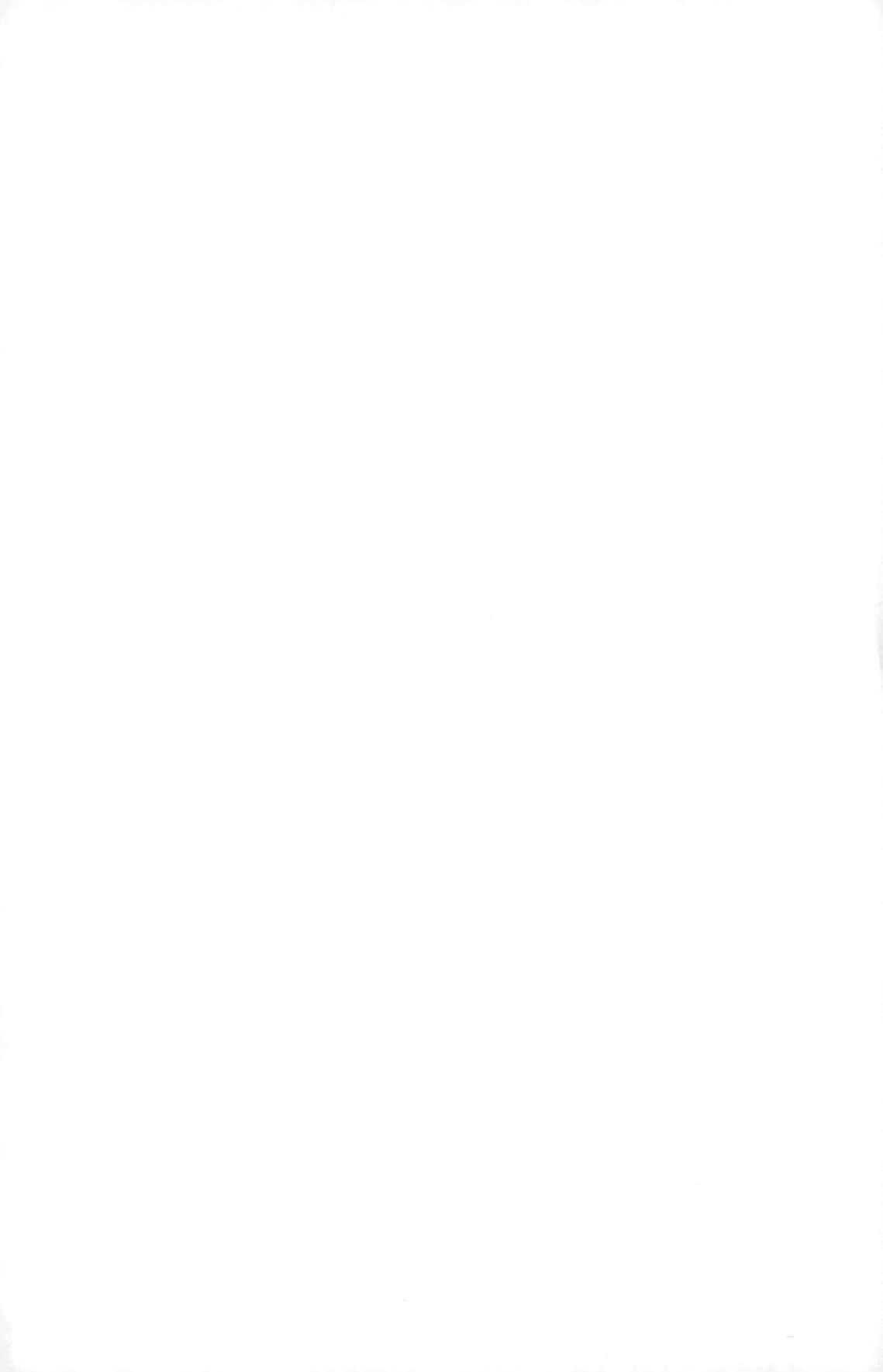

www.ingramcontent.com/pod-product-compliance
Ingram Content Group UK Ltd.
Pitfield, Milton Keynes, MK11 3LW, UK
UKHW022153230426
12049UKWH00003BA/80